Portal Hypertension - Recent Advances

Edited by Xingshun Qi

Published in London, United Kingdom

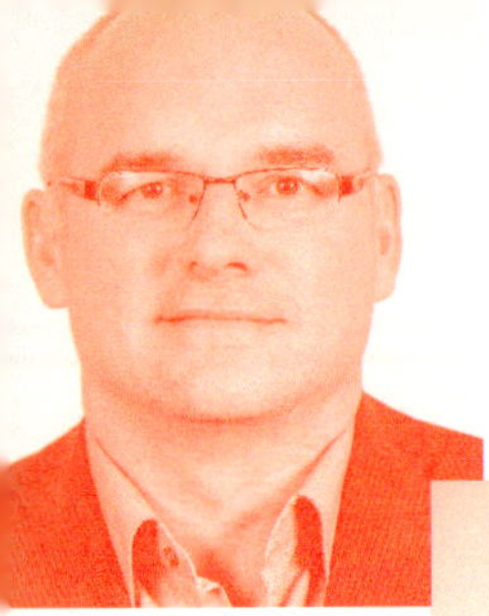
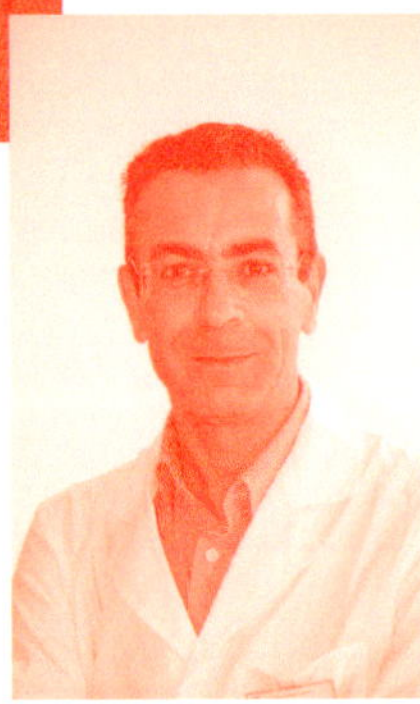
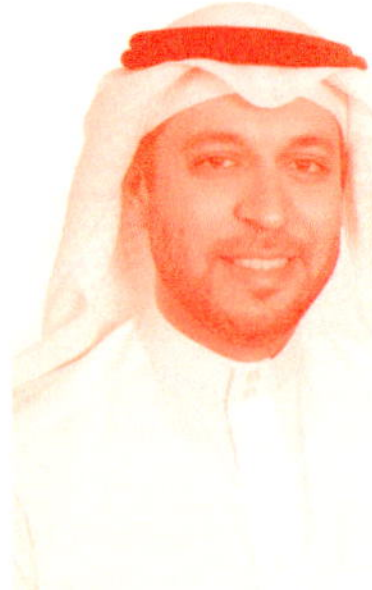
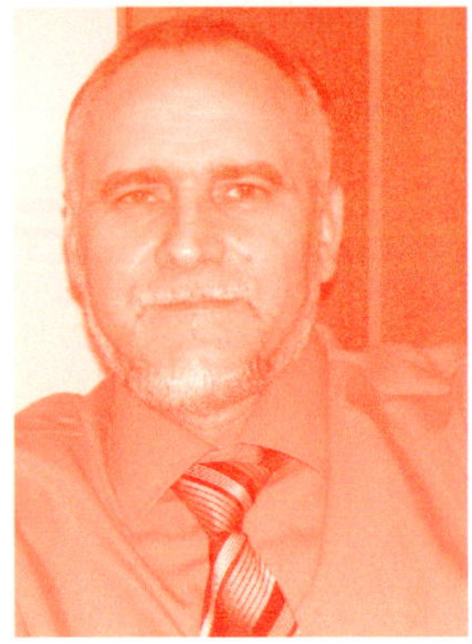
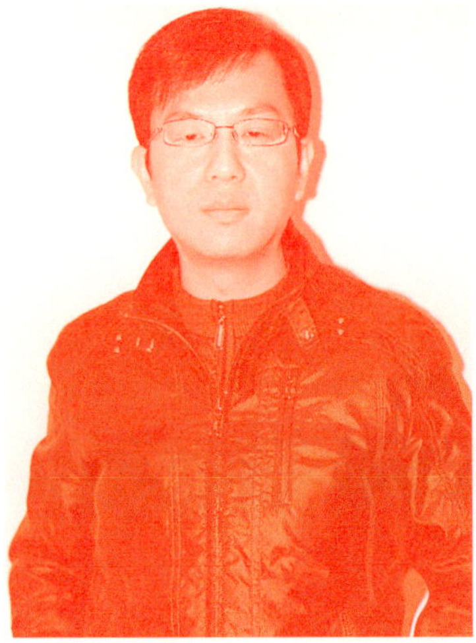
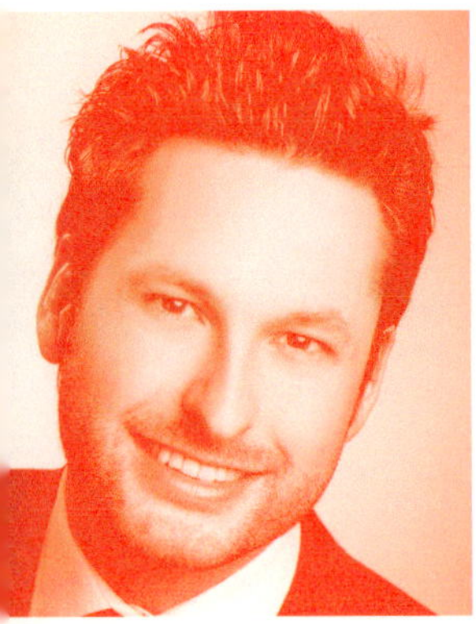
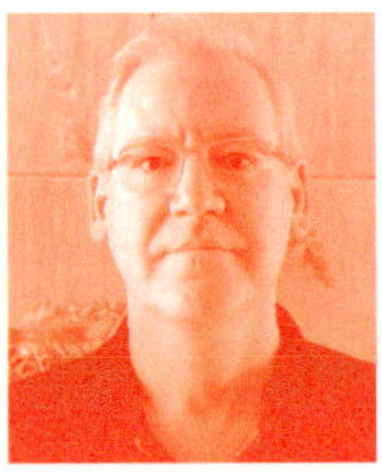

IntechOpen

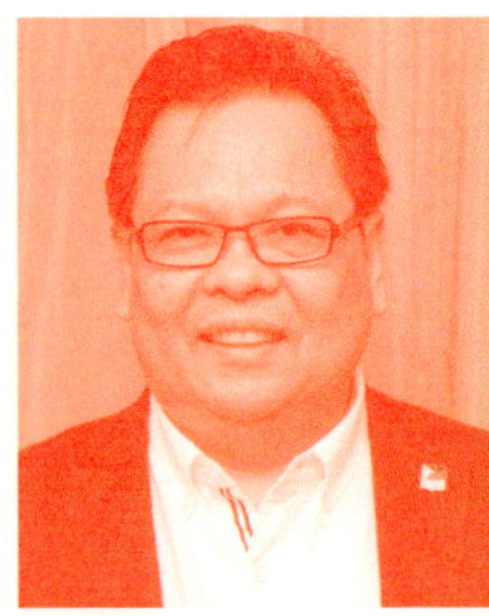
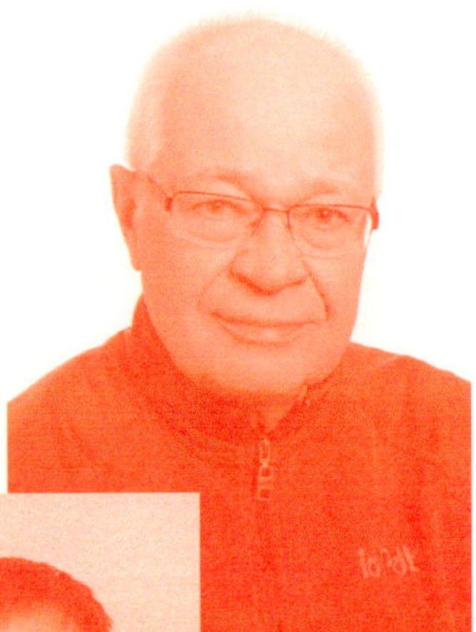
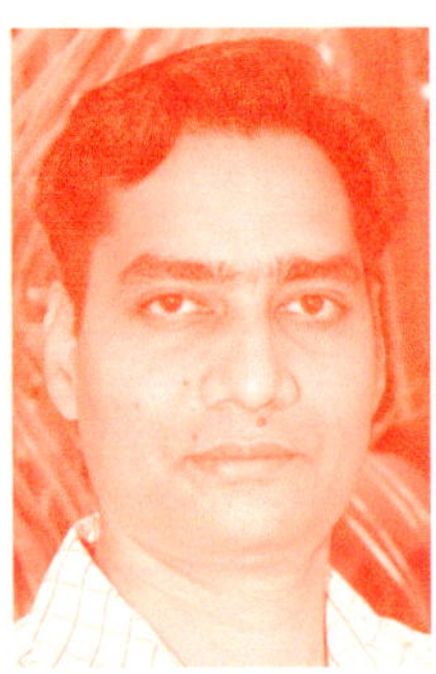
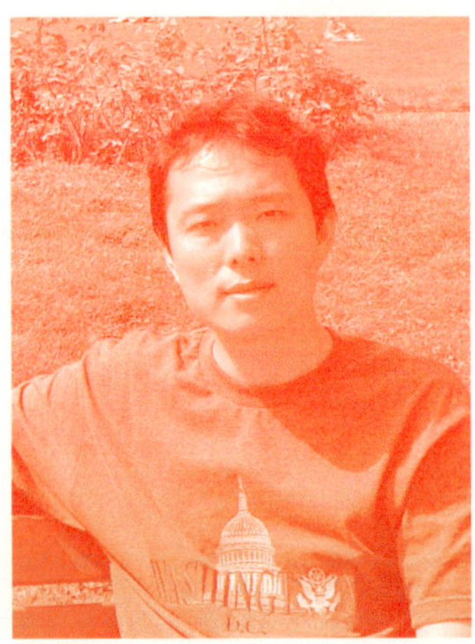
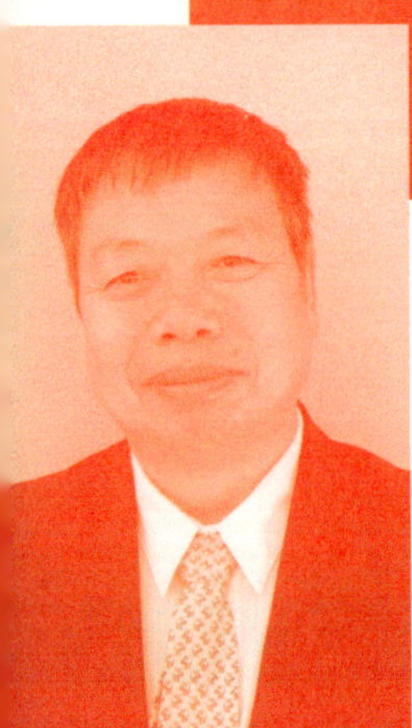
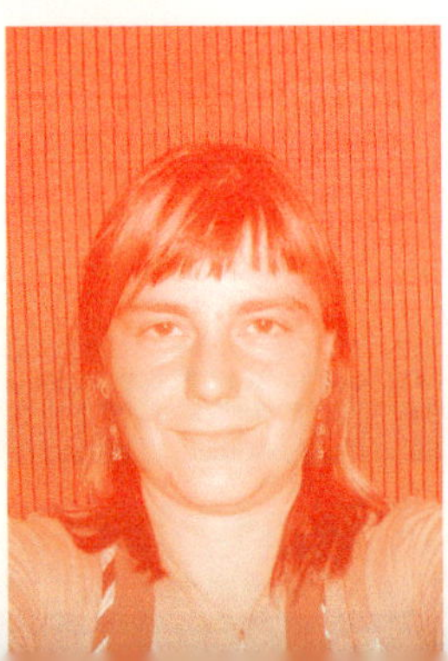

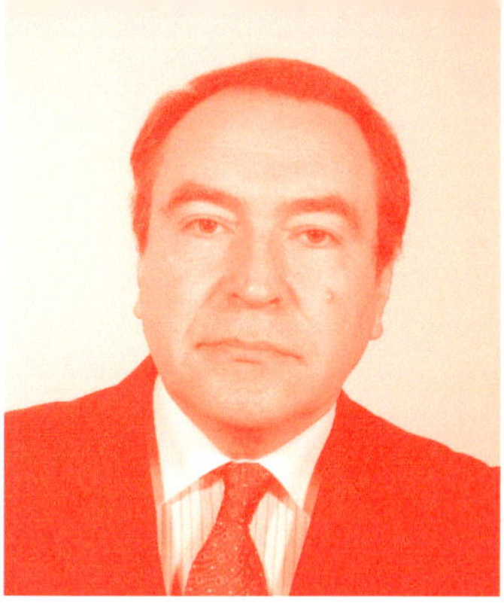
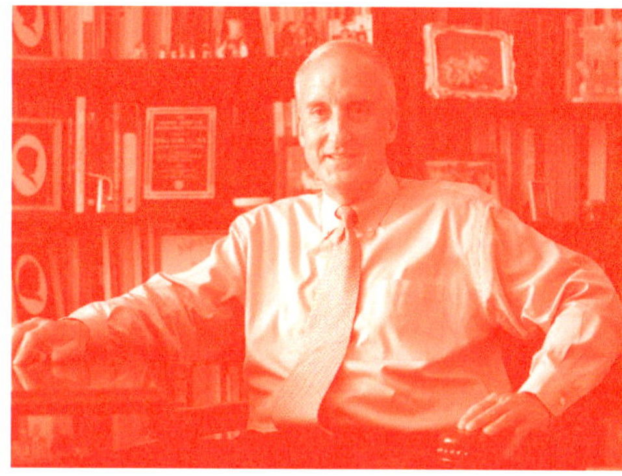
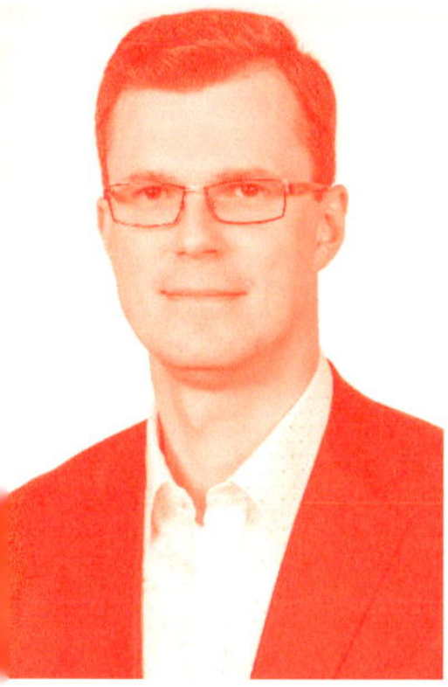
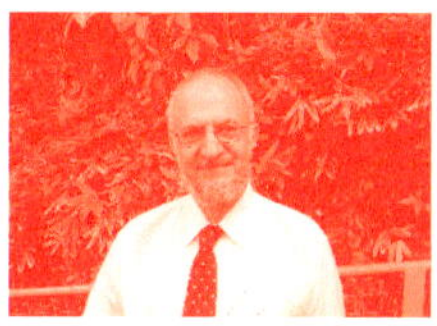
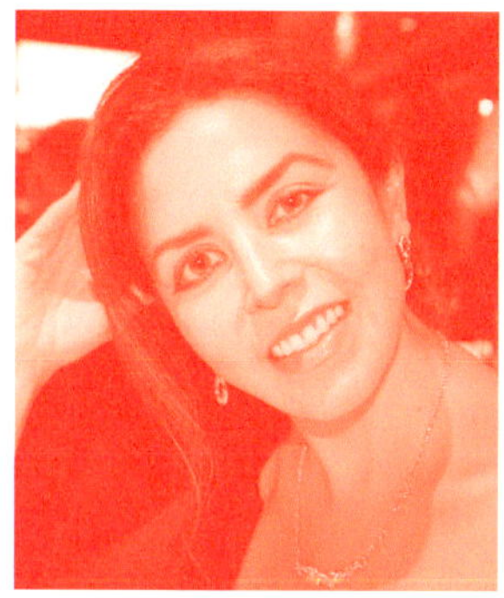

Supporting open minds since 2005

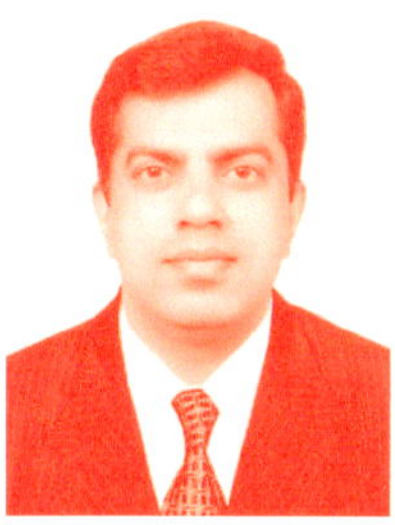
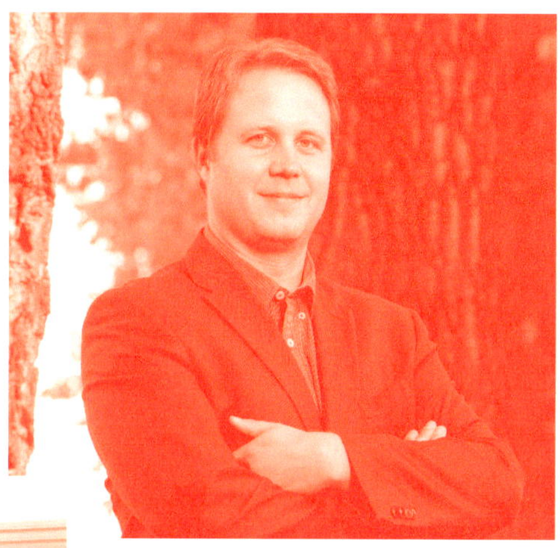
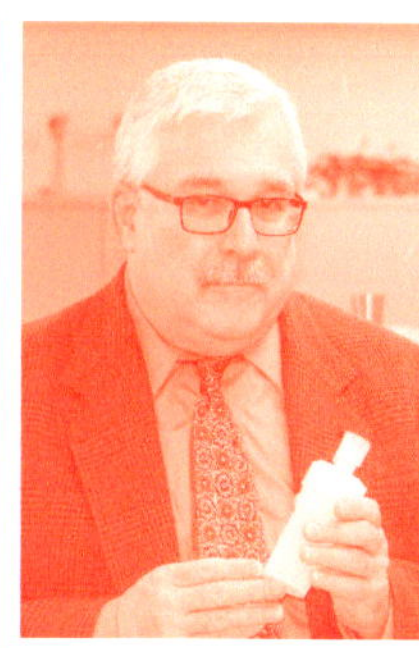
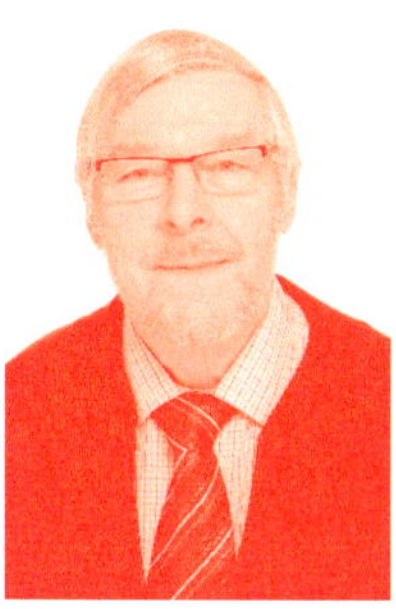
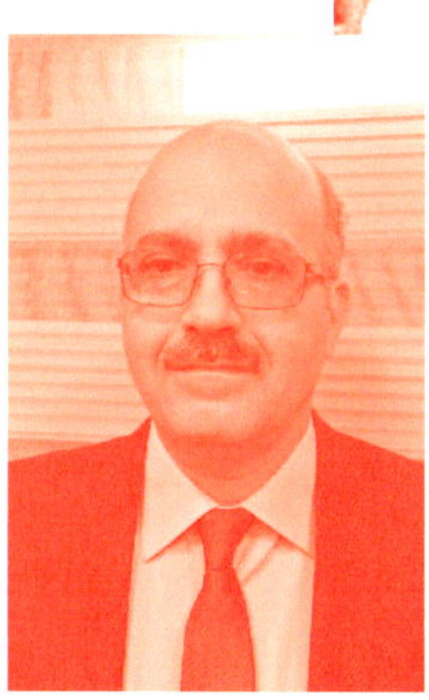
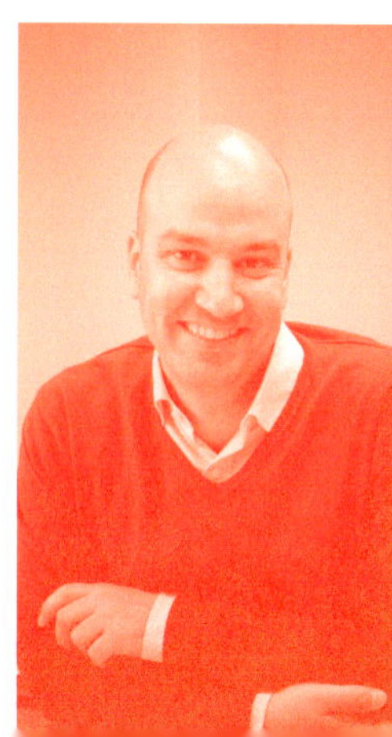
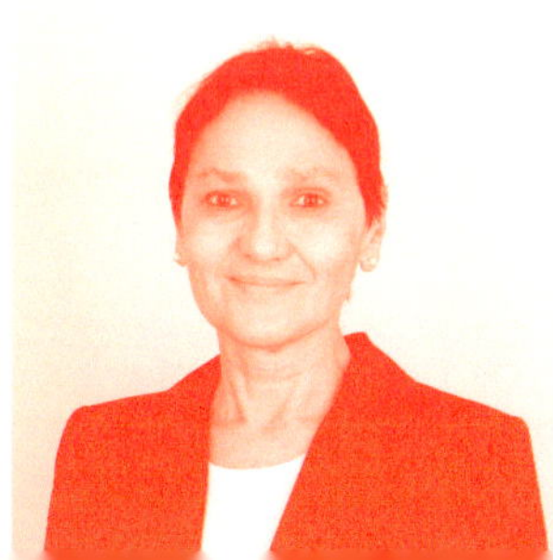

Portal Hypertension - Recent Advances
http://dx.doi.org/10.5772/intechopen.91608
Edited by Xingshun Qi

Contributors
Mahesh Goenka, Bhavik Shah, Usha Goenka, Jinfeng Yang, Shuangfa Zou, Peng Yanhua, Zhen Chumeng, Yanxia Fei, Huiping Sun, Achyut Bikram Hamal, Reda Zbaida, Elena Curakova Ristovska, Xingshun Qi, Ran Wang, Xiaozhong Guo

First published in London, United Kingdom, 2021 by IntechOpen
IntechOpen is the global imprint of INTECHOPEN LIMITED, registered in England and Wales, registration number: 11086078, 5 Princes Gate Court, London, SW7 2QJ, United Kingdom
Printed in Croatia

British Library Cataloguing-in-Publication Data
A catalogue record for this book is available from the British Library

Additional hard and PDF copies can be obtained from orders@intechopen.com

Portal Hypertension - Recent Advances
Edited by Xingshun Qi
p. cm.
Print ISBN 978-1-83968-343-5
Online ISBN 978-1-83968-344-2
eBook (PDF) ISBN 978-1-83968-359-6

For EU product safety concerns:
IN TECH d.o.o., Prolaz Marije Krucifikse Kozulić 3, 51000 Rijeka, Croatia, info@intechopen.com or visit our website at intechopen.com.

Meet the editor

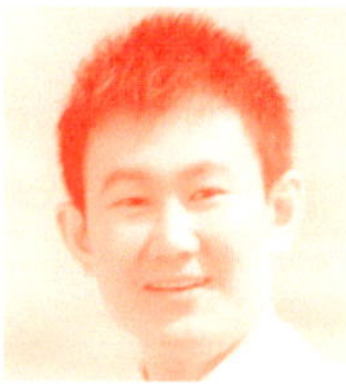

Dr. Xingshun Qi obtained his medical doctoral degree at the Fourth Military Medical University and completed his post-doctoral fellowship at the General Hospital of Shenyang Military Area, China. Currently, he is a deputy director at the Department of Gastroenterology at General Hospital of Northern Theater Command (formerly General Hospital of Shenyang Military Area). His major research interests are the management of liver cirrhosis, portal hypertension (especially portal vein thrombosis and Budd-Chiari syndrome), and hepatocellular carcinoma. He has edited six English-language books and serves as an associate editor for *BMC Gastroenterology*, an academic editor for the *Canadian Journal of Gastroenterology and Hepatology*, and an advisory editorial member of *Advances in Therapy*. His H-index is 37 with 4467 citations to date.

Contents

Preface

Portal hypertension is a rise in the pressure gradient between the portal vein and the inferior vena cava. Realistically, it is difficult to directly measure the portal vein pressure. For this reason, hepatic venous pressure gradient, which can be calculated by subtracting wedged hepatic vein pressure from free hepatic vein pressure, has been employed in clinical practice to establish a diagnosis of portal hypertension. There are various types of portal hypertension, including pre-hepatic, hepatic, and post-hepatic. Nowadays, the management of portal hypertension and its complications is still a clinical challenge.

This book, *Portal Hypertension - Recent Advances* does not intend to cover all areas of management of portal hypertension, but rather focuses on the recent advances in several major topics, including pediatric portal hypertension, sinusoidal obstructions syndrome, endoscopy in the management of portal hypertension, and non-invasive assessment of esophageal varices. These topics should be interesting and helpful for gastroenterologists, hepatologists, endoscopists, and pediatricians interested in this field.

Finally, I greatly appreciate the contributions from the chapter authors and the assistance from Josip Knapić, Author Service Manager at IntechOpen.

Xingshun Qi
Department of Gastroenterology,
General Hospital of Northern Theater Command,
Shenyang, China

Section 1

Overviews of Portal Hypertension

Chapter 1

Brief Review of Portal Hypertension Related Complications

Achyut Bikram Hamal

Abstract

The pathologic increase in the pressure gradient between portal vein and inferior venacava is called portal hypertension. Increased portal blood flow and increased resistance in the portal venous system cause portal hypertension. The structural components and the functional components contribute to the resistance. Hepatic venous pressure gradient (HVPG) reflects the degree of portal pressure in liver disease. HVPG is calculated as the difference between the wedged hepatic venous pressure (WHVP) and the free hepatic venous pressure (FHVP). Clinically significant portal hypertension (CSPH) is defined as HVPG $\geq$10. Different values of HVPG have been defined as threshold for different consequences of portal hypertension. Variceal hemorrhage, portal hypertensive gastropathy, ascites, colopathy, biliopathy and hepatopulmonary syndrome are main complications of portal hypertension. Besides nonselective beta blockers, other drugs like statins, antioxidants, antidiabetic, anti-inflammatory and antiapoptotic drugs have also been seen to be effective in reducing portal pressure.

Keywords: portal hypertension, Hepatic venous pressure gradient (HVPG), variceal hemorrhage, hepatopulmonary syndrome, cirrhotic cardiomyopathy

1. Introduction

Vesalius [1] was the person who drew an anatomical picture of the portal venous system in 1543 and described a case of bleeding hemorrhoids and suggested that this was due to a dilatation of the portal branches. Glisson [2] at a dissection in London, in 1650 established that blood was collected from the gastrointestinal tract by portal vein and finally to the systemic circulation.

Morgagni described a patient who had died from gastrointestinal hemorrhage: at the autopsy, dilatation of the splenic vein and of the short gastric veins were found.

The name cirrhosis was introduced in 1819, in Paris, by Renè Laennec, deriving from two words of the antique Greek: Skirros (hard, fibrotic) and Kirrhos (yellowish). He used the word "cirrhosis" in the textbook published by him [3].

Dusaussey [4], wrote an important thesis 'Studies on esophageal varices in liver cirrhosis', in 1872. He believed that the obstruction to portal flow was a consequence of liver cirrhosis.

Gilbert [5] introduced the term portal hypertension in 1902. A 'pressure close to that in the portal vein' without opening the abdomen, was obtained by puncturing one of the dilated abdominal wall veins (the caput medusae) by Davidson [6].

Thompson (1937) [7] directly measured portal pressure for the first time, with the open abdomen, the pressure in the portal vein and in the inferior vena cava. In 1953 Lebon et al. [8] diagnosed portal hypertension by percutaneous measurement of the intrasplenic pressure.

2. Definition

Patients with portal hypertension are identified when they present to hospitals or clinic after they have complications such as ascites, gastrointestinal bleeding, hepatic encephalopathy or hypersplenism. The pressure gradient between the portal vein and the inferior vena cava (the so-called portal perfusion pressure of the liver or portal pressure gradient) increases to greater than the normal range of values (1–5 mm Hg) when there is pathologic increase in portal pressure, which is called portal hypertension [9].

3. Portal pressure measurement and its importance

While evaluating them the need for the evaluating the underlying cirrhosis, the degree of portal hypertension, the site of obstruction and the presence of collateral circulation makes the diagnosis of portal hypertension complete [10]. As the disease progresses, the amount of fibrosis increases and in parallel the portal pressure rises corresponding to worsening in the prognosis. Direct or indirect measurement of portal pressure can be done with various methods.

Measurement of the hepatic venous pressure gradient (HVPG) is the gold standard technique used to quantify the degree portal hypertension in liver disease. Diagnosis, classification, and monitoring of portal hypertension, risk stratification, identification of candidates for liver resection, and monitoring efficacy of β-adrenergic blockers are the main clinical applications of HVPG measurements.

HVPG is calculated as the difference between the wedged hepatic venous pressure (WHVP) and the free hepatic venous pressure (FHVP) [11]. The WHVP is measured by occluding a main hepatic vein which causes the static column of blood to transmit the pressure that is present in the preceding vascular territory i. e. the hepatic sinusoids. This measurement, in the absence of presinusoidal obstruction, reflects portal pressure [12]. The FHVP is a measure of the pressure of unoccluded hepatic vein. HVPG calculated with right atrial pressure shows a worse correlation with clinical outcomes, therefore FHVP should be used [13]. There are several methods to measure portal pressure as enumerated in **Table 1**.

The changes in HVPG are due to the alterations in the intrahepatic resistance, collateral resistance, portal blood inflow or their combination [14]. Dynamic factors such as hepatic vascular tone and mechanical factors such as fibrosis, thrombosis and formation of regenerative nodules cause the alterations in HVPG.

The complications of portal hypertension increase as HVPG increases. Clinical manifestations and complications occur at a threshold of HVPG of 10 mm Hg, which is called clinically significant portal hypertension (CSPH). Different thresholds of HVPG correlate with different prognostic significance (**Table 2**).

3.1 Technique of measurement of HVPG

Under sedation a balloon-tipped catheter is introduced through the central line inserted into the right internal jugular vein, usually under ultrasound guidance [28].

SN	Methods	Procedures
1.	Indirect estimation of Portal hypertension	Ascitic fluid analysis Serum Ascitic Albumin Gradient (SAAG) ≥ 1.1
2.	Hepatic Vein Pressure Gradient (HVPG)	Open-ended catheter placed in one of the hepatic veins via a supraclavicular or internal jugular approach. Double-lumen balloon catheter placed in the hepatic vein via a femoral approach
3.	Direct measurement of the portal pressure gradient	The portal vein can be catheterized directly, either by a trans hepatic approach or by a catheter placed via the umbilical vein. The added advantage is that collaterals can be embolized while this procedure. Angiography can be performed at the same time to minimize the number of procedures performed. Portal pressure measurements should be obtained prior to the injection of contrast, which in itself can alter pressures.
4.	Intrahepatic portal vein pressure	Percutaneous catheterization of an intrahepatic branch of the portal vein with a thin Chiba needle; a catheter is passed via the intrahepatic branch into the main portal vein.
5.	Intrasplenic pressure	Placement of a needle percutaneously in the substance of the spleen.
6.	Umbilical vein catheter	Requires dissection to expose the umbilical vein; may require dilation of the umbilical vein to facilitate advancement of the catheter.

Table 1.
Different methods of measuring portal pressure.

HVPG	Clinical characteristics
< 5 mm Hg	Normal
5–10 mm Hg	Mild portal hypertension
>6 mm Hg	Progression of chronic viral hepatitis [15]
	High risk of recurrence after liver transplantation [16]
>10 mm Hg	Clinically significant Portal hypertension (CSPH)
>10 mm Hg	Esophageal variceal development [17, 18]
	Decompensation with ascites [19]
	Hepatocellular carcinoma (HCC) [20]
	Decompensation after Hepatic resection [21]
>12 mm Hg	Variceal bleeding [22, 23]
>16 mm Hg	High mortality [24]
>20 mm Hg	Failure to control bleeding in acute variceal bleed [25] Low 1-year survival
>22 mm Hg	High mortality in severe alcoholic hepatitis [26]
>30 mm Hg	Spontaneous bacterial peritonitis (SBP) [27]

Table 2.
Different thresholds of hepatic venous pressure gradient (HVPG) correlated with prognostic significance.

The catheter is advanced through the right atrium into the inferior venacava (IVC) under fluoroscopic guidance and then pushed into the right hepatic vein. Alternatively, the femoral approach can be used.

FHVP is obtained after the catheter is maintained in the hepatic vein 2 to 4 cm from its takeoff from the IVC. Typically, the difference in pressure between the IVC (measured at the hepatic vein ostium) and hepatic vein is ≤1 mmHg. If the difference is >1 mmHg it means the catheter is placed too deep into the hepatic vein. After this, WHVP is measured after the hepatic vein is occluded by inflating the balloon at the tip of the catheter. A small amount of contrast dye (5 mL) or carbon dioxide (if allergic to the contrast) is injected to confirm that the hepatic vein is occluded so that no reflux of the dye above the balloon or should washout via communications with other hepatic veins. Around 3 each measurements of wedged and free hepatic venous pressure are made each time with the stability of the value for at least 45–60 seconds [29]. Finally, the HVPG is calculated by subtracting the FHVP from the WHVP.

The findings of hemodynamic measurements in patients with intrahepatic portal hypertension are enumerated [28] in **Table 3**.

At the same time along with HVPG measurement include transjugular liver biopsy, measurement of hepatic blood flow and indocyanine green clearance, and wedged hepatic retrograde portography using carbon dioxide can be done. Complications during the procedure can be arrhythmia or injury to the local site.

3.2 Noninvasive tests

Though these noninvasive tests cannot replace HVPG measurement for confirming the diagnosis of portal hypertension, ultrasonogram and transient elastography may be helpful.

3.2.1 Ultrasonography

Portal hypertension findings in transabdominal ultrasound are [28]:

- Ascites
- Splenomegaly (> 13 cm or Splenic index >20 cm^2)
- Coarse echotexture of liver with irregular margin and dull edge
- Portal flow mean velocity < 12 cm/second
- Reversal of flow in the portal vein and left gastric vein
- Portosystemic collaterals (patent-paraumbilical vein, splenorenal collaterals, dilated left and short gastric veins)
- Portal vein diameter > 13 mm
- Decreased or no respiratory variation in splenic and superior mesenteric vein diameter
- Portal/splenic/superior mesenteric vein thrombosis

Hemodynamic measurement	Presinusoidal	Sinusoidal	Post-sinusoidal
FHVP (a)	Normal	Sinusoidal	Increased
WHVP (b)	Normal or mild increased	Increased	Increased
HVPG (b-a)	Normal or mild increased	Increased	Normal

Table 3.
Hemodynamic measurements in portal hypertension.

3.2.2 Transient elastography

Transient elastography using ultrasound is a noninvasive method for detecting hepatic fibrosis. Studies are also looking at it as an option for noninvasively diagnosing portal hypertension.

A value <13.6 kPa can be used to rule out portal hypertension, whereas a value ≥21.1 kPa is likely to have portal hypertension [28].

4. Pathophysiology of portal hypertension

With the concept of physics, it is important to note that portal hypertension is related to both flow and resistance.

Pressure (P) equals flow (Q) times resistance (R), demonstrated by the formula.

$$P = Q \times R$$

Resistance is a function of the length and radius as shown by the formula R = 8n L/IIr^4, where n is the coefficient of viscosity, L is the length of the vessel, and r is the radius. The pathophysiology of portal hypertension is explained in **Figure 1**.

4.1 Etiology of portal hypertension

Various etiologies of portal hypertension can be enumerated as:

Prehepatic
Splenic vein thrombosis
Portal vein thrombosis
Congenital portal vein stenosis
Cavernomatosis of the portal vein
Arteriovenous fistula
Tropical splenomegaly
Intrahepatic
Presinusoidal: Schistosomiasis
Sarcoidosis
Primary Biliary Cirrhosis (Early)
Chronic active hepatitis
Congenital hepatic fibrosis
Hepatic artery portal vein fistula
Porto-sclerosis
Drugs
Arsenic, copper sulfate and Vinyl chloride poisoning.
Amyloidosis
Tuberculosis
Wilsons disease
Hemochromatosis
Mastocytosis
Sinusoidal: Acute alcoholic Hepatitis
Liver cirrhosis independent of etiology
Amyloidosis
Partial nodular transformation
Nodular regenerative hyperplasia
Hypervitaminosis A

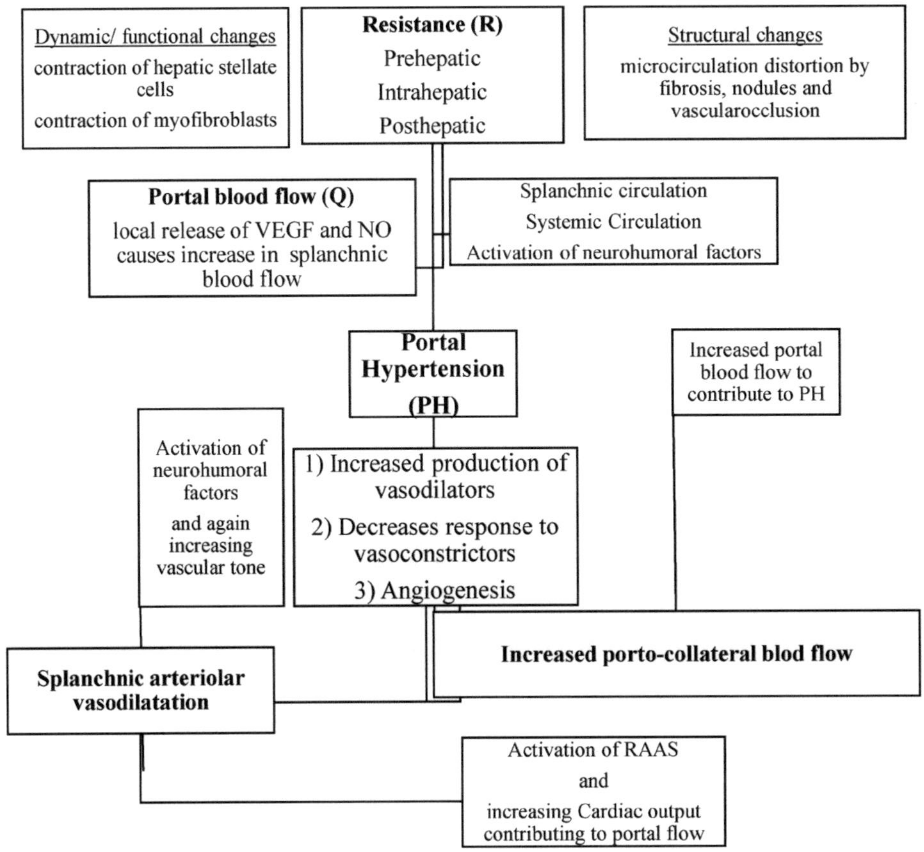

Figure 1.
Pathophysiology of portal hypertension.

Cytotoxic drugs
Acute fatty liver of pregnancy
Peliosis hepatitis
Polycystic liver disease
Idiopathic portal hypertension
Metastatic malignant disease
Post-sinusoidal: Veno-occlusive disease
Alcoholic central hyaline sclerosis
Post-hepatic
Budd-Chiari syndrome
Congenital malformations and thrombosis of the inferior vena cava
Constrictive pericarditis
Congenital heart diseases
Cardiomyopathy
Tricuspid valve diseases
Miscellaneous
Arteriovenous fistulas (splenic, aorto-mesenteric, aorto-portal, and hepatic artery-portal vein)

Formation of collateral circulation connects the portal blood vessels to systemic circulation, bypassing the liver and leading to portal hypertension [30]. Sometimes, when a pathological process causes occlusion of the splenic vein and the resultant elevated splenic bed venous pressure causes formation of gastric varices which can lead to hematemesis it is called sinistral portal hypertension. Sinistral portal hypertension is a rare, less than 1%, but life-threatening cause of upper gastric bleeding. In fact, the name sinistral portal hypertension is a misnomer since portal pressure is usually within the normal range in these cases. Other names for sinistral portal hypertension are left sided portal hypertension, segmental, regional, localized, compartmental, lineal, or spleno-portal hypertension [31–33]. It accounts for less than 5% of all patients with portal hypertension [33].

Chronic pancreatitis, pancreatic cancer, pancreatic cysts and neuroendocrine tumor are common causes of sinistral portal hypertension. Most involved vessel in pancreatitis-related splanchnic vein thrombosis is splenic vein followed by portal vein and mesenteric vein. It is mainly related to pancreatic inflammation and compression by pancreatic pseudocyst [34]. Around 8% of patients of chronic pancreatitis experience splenic vein thrombosis, the majority do not experience any form of symptomatic GI bleeding [35]. They present with hypersplenism, abdominal pain and gastrointestinal bleeding. They should undergo gastroscopy evaluation in search of varices. Suspicion of this portal hypertension should be done when patient has gastric varices only in fundus with or without any aberrant liver functions or features of liver cirrhosis with the presence of splenomegaly.

Iatrogenic splenic vein injury, ectopic spleen, colonic tumor infiltration, peri-renal abscess, post liver transplantation, Hodgkin's disease, retro-peritoneal fibrosis, pancreatic transplantation, and spontaneous thrombus formation are among the less common causes of splenic vein thrombosis that can lead to left sided hypertension [31, 32].

5. Complications of portal hypertension

Patients with portal hypertension are usually asymptomatic until they develop complications. Complications of portal hypertension include:

1. Variceal hemorrhage
2. Portal hypertensive gastropathy (PHG)
3. Ascites
4. Spontaneous bacterial peritonitis
5. Hepatorenal syndrome (HRS)
6. Hepatic hydrothorax
7. Hepatopulmonary syndrome (HPS)
8. Porto-pulmonary hypertension (POPH)
9. Portal hypertensive colopathy
10. Cirrhotic cardiomyopathy
11. Portal Biliopathy

5.1 Variceal hemorrhage

Bleeding occurs in 30%–40% of patients with cirrhosis and varices [36]. The incidence of first variceal bleeding is about 12–15% per year in patients with cirrhosis and esophageal varices and mortality ranges from 17% - 57% in patients at first episode of variceal bleeding [37]. Carbonell et al. has also estimated mortality during the first episode of bleeding to be 15–20% but with Child Pugh C, it is around 30% [38].

The preventive measures advocated are beta blockers and endoscopic variceal ligation (EVL). Beta blockers provide protection against rebleeding after index hemorrhage while local obliteration of varices is done by EVL.

Nonselective beta blockers have been used daily in patients with cirrhosis and portal hypertension with varices either for primary or secondary prophylaxis. Recommended agents for primary prophylaxis of variceal hemorrhage are propranolol and nadolol [39, 40].

Secondary prophylaxis with nonspecific beta blocker (NSBB) has been shown to be effective in decreasing both the risk of recurrent bleeding and mortality [41, 42]. Without secondary prophylaxis, rebleeding occurs in approximately 60% to 70% of patients, usually within one to two years of the index hemorrhagic event [43]. Most used NSBB for secondary prophylaxis is propranolol but carvedilol can also be used. The decrease in HR at 6 weeks was significantly higher in carvedilol than propranolol group ($p = 0.036$). The rebleeding at least once within 6 months was also higher in propranolol group than carvedilol group (32 vs. 22.7%) [44].

5.2 Portal hypertensive Gastropathy

It is the characteristic appearance which is a mosaic-like pattern or a diffuse, erythematous and reticular cobblestone pattern of gastric mucosa consisting of small polygonal areas, with or without superimposed red punctate lesions, >2 mm in diameter and a depressed white border [45–47]. PHG is classified as mild or severe.

Mild PHG has features like fine pink speckling (scarlatina-type rash), and mosaic pattern (snakeskin appearance) and Severe one has discrete red spots or diffuse hemorrhagic lesion [48].

The prevalence of PHG in Nepalese population with Chronic Liver Diseases (CLD) was 67 percent [49] though it varies significantly from 16 to 100 percentage [50]. Acute bleeding in PHG is estimated to occur in 2 to 12 percent [51].

5.3 Ascites

Patients with cirrhosis with portal hypertension may present with ascites leading to distension of abdomen and dyspnea. They will have flank fullness with dullness on examination. The grading of ascites as graded by International Club for Ascites are [52]:

- Grade 1 – Mild ascites detectable only by ultrasound examination
- Grade 2 – Moderate ascites manifested by moderate symmetrical distension of the abdomen
- Grade 3 – Large or gross ascites with marked abdominal distension

Ascites may range from mild to refractory. Mild to moderate ascites should be managed by modest salt restriction and combination of loop diuretics and potassium sparing diuretics.

Ultrasonographic detection of mild ascites is either pelvic or perihepatic or peri splenic ascites, while moderate ascites is presence of pelvic and perihepatic and perisplenic ascites, and marked ascites is diffuse ascites in the peritoneal cavity [52].

Diuretics should be added in a stepwise fashion along with sodium restriction. Gross ascites should be treated with therapeutic paracentesis followed by colloid volume expansion, and diuretic therapy. Sometimes refractory ascites is managed by repeated large volume paracentesis or insertion of a transjugular intrahepatic portosystemic stent shunt (TIPS) [53].

5.4 Spontaneous bacterial peritonitis (SBP)

Spontaneous bacterial peritonitis occurs with a prevalence of 10–25% in cirrhotic patients with ascites [54]. It can be community acquired, health care associated or nosocomial.

Major pathogenic organisms are *E. coli* (24.3%), followed by *Klebsiella pneumoniae* (12.0%) and *Enterococcus faecium* (10.5%). Nosocomial SBP has significantly higher proportion of Enterococcus (27.7% vs. 6.1%, $P < 0.001$) than community acquired SBP. Nosocomial SBP has a poorer outcome than community acquired pneumonia (24.6% vs. 36.8%; $P = 0.016$). The independent predictors for 30-day mortality are nosocomial infection, Child-Pugh classification, hepatocellular carcinoma, renal failure and hepatic encephalopathy [54].

Suspicion of nosocomial SBP should be done in a patient with SBP with a history of ICU stay during the previous 3 months or on prophylactic antibiotics for infection or had antibiotic treatment during previous 3 months or had a recent intervention in the hospital setting. Resistance to 3rd generation cephalosporins and quinolones has been documented in 40–50% of such cases [55].

Recently, Elsadek et al. found that Patients with SBP ($n = 60$) have significantly higher serum PEC index than those with sterile ascites ($n = 118$) (41.0/31.2–93.0 vs. 9.9/5.9–15.0, $P < 0.001$) and it distinguished culture positive cases significantly ($P < 0.001$) [56].

Diagnostic paracentesis should be performed in all patients who present with [57] (1) compatible signs or symptoms (abdominal pain and/or tenderness on palpation, fever, and chills); (2) impairment of the hepatic or renal function; (3) unexplained hepatic encephalopathy; (4) gastrointestinal bleeding.

SBP is diagnosed by polymorphonuclear cells ≥250 cells/mm^3 in ascitic fluid in the absence of an intra-abdominal and surgically treatable source of infection. Other potential diagnostic methods are leukocyte esterase reagent strips (LERS), measurement of leukocyte-derived proteins such as granulocyte elastase and lactoferrin, detection of bacterial DNA using polymerase chain reaction (PCR) and detecting bacterial DNA in SBP ascites using in situ hybridization [57].

5.5 Hepatorenal syndrome (HRS)

HRS occurs in the setting of advanced cirrhosis and portal hypertension [58] with prevalence of 13–45 percentage [59]. It is characterized by peripheral arterial vasodilatation and intrarenal vasoconstriction with decrease in renal blood flow and renal dysfunction. The most recent proposed diagnostic criteria for HRS-AKI are as-.

Diagnostic Criteria for HRS-AKI [60].

- Cirrhosis with ascites; acute liver failure; acute-on-chronic liver failure

- Increase in serum creatinine ≥0.3 mg/dl within 48 h or ≥ 50% from baseline value according to International Club of Ascites (ICA) consensus document and/or urinary output ≤0.5 ml/kg B.W. ≥ 6 h*

- No full or partial response, according to the ICA consensus, after at least 2 days of diuretic withdrawal and volume expansion with albumin. The recommended dose of albumin is 1 gm/kg of body weight per day to a maximum of 100 gm/day

- Absence of shock

- No current or recent treatment with nephrotoxic drugs

- Absence of parenchymal disease as indicated by proteinuria >500 mg/day, micro-hematuria (>50 red blood cells per high power field), urinary injury biomarkers (if available) and/or abnormal renal ultrasonography**.

- Suggestion of renal vasoconstriction with FENa of <0.2% (with levels <0.1% being highly predictive)

*The evaluation of this parameter requires a urinary catheter.

**This criterion would not be included in cases of known pre-existing structural chronic kidney disease (e. g. diabetic or hypertensive nephropathy). AKI, acute kidney injury; FENa, fractional excretion of sodium; HRS, hepatorenal syndrome.

Nowadays, HRS has been classified as HRS-AKI and HRS-NAKI. The diagnosis.

of HRS-NAKI has been proposed to be made in the context of CKD, or AKD that does not meet the criteria for AKI and lasts for <90 days.

HRS-AKD is defined as a percent increase in sCr <50% or as an eGFR <60 min/ml per 1.73 m2 for <3 months with the fulfillment of the ICA criteria for HRS.

HRS-CKD defined as an eGFR <60 ml/min per 1.73 m2 for ≥3 months with the fulfillment of the ICA criteria.

Treatment can be done with terlipressin with albumin as medical treatment or with liver transplantation.

5.6 Hepatic hydrothorax

Hepatic hydrothorax (HH) is defined as the excessive (> 500 mL) accumulation of transudate fluid in the pleural cavity in patients with decompensated liver cirrhosis (LC) with exclusion of cardiopulmonary and pleural diseases [61]. It is present in 5–10% of cirrhotic patients. Right sided HH is common accounting for almost 85% of cases followed by left sided (13%). The mechanism of HH is due to negative intrathoracic pressure and liver acting as piston which results the ascitic fluid to move from the peritoneal cavity into the pleural space through small defects located mainly on the right side of the diaphragmatic tendon [61, 62]. Huang et al. [63] classified diaphragmatic defects into four types: (1) Type 1 - no obvious defects; (2) Type 2 – blebs lying on the diaphragm; (3) Type 3 – broken defects (fenestrations) in the diaphragm; (4) Type 4 – multiple gaps in the diaphragm.

The diagnostic criteria [61] for HH are listed in **Table 4**.

The options for treatment for refractory HH are low sodium diet with therapeutic thoracocentesis, pleurodesis, mesh repair of diaphragmatic defects, transjugular

Criteria	Values
Count of white blood cells in pleural fluid	< 250/mm^3
Pleural effusion total protein level	< 25 g/L
Pleural effusion total protein/serum total protein ratio	< 0.5
Pleural effusion Lactate dehydrogenase (LDH)/serum LDH ratio	> 0.6
Pleural effusion albumin/serum albumin ratio	> 1.1
Pleural effusion bilirubin /serum bilirubin ratio	< 0.6
pH	> 7.4
Pleural effusion glucose level is equal to serum glucose level	

Table 4.
The diagnostic criteria for hepatic hydrothorax.

intrahepatic portosystemic shunt (TIPS), pleuro-venous or peritoneo-venous shunting though liver transplantation is the definite therapy.

5.7 Hepato-pulmonary syndrome (HPS)

HPS is defined as a disorder in pulmonary oxygenation, caused by intrapulmonary. vasodilatation and, less commonly, by pleural and pulmonary arteriovenous communications occurring in the clinical setting of portal hypertension. HPS has been reported in 10% of patients with chronic viral hepatitis in 15–23% of those with cirrhosis and in 28% of those with Budd-Chiari syndrome [64].

The diagnostic criteria for HPS are [64]:

1. Hypoxia with partial pressure of oxygen <80 mmHg or alveolar–arterial oxygen gradient ≥15 mmHg in ambient air (≥20 mmHg in patients older than 65 years).

2. Pulmonary vascular defect with positive findings on contrast-enhanced echocardiography (i.e., microbubble opacification of the left heart chambers three to six cycles after right atrial passage) or abnormal uptake in the brain (>6%) with radioactive lung-perfusion scanning.

Spontaneous resolution of HPS is less likely and the definite treatment is liver transplantation however long-term oxygen therapy remains the most frequently recommended therapy for symptoms in patients with severe hypoxaemia. No established medical therapy is found however some improvement in Pao2 with garlic has been seen [65].

5.8 Portopulmonary syndrome (POPH)

Vasoconstriction, vascular remodeling, and proliferative and thrombotic events within the pulmonary circulation lead to POPH. The presence of portal hypertension, hemodynamic measurements of mean pulmonary artery pressure > 25 mmHg at rest, mean pulmonary capillary wedge pressure < 15 mmHg, and pulmonary vascular resistance >240 dynes/cm^{-5} confirm POPH [66].

POPH is commonly diagnosed during fifth decade of life, 4–7 years after the presence of portal hypertension has been established [67]. Symptoms include dyspnea, fatigue, light headedness, and orthopnea in patients with liver cirrhosis or portal hypertension. Diuretics can be used for symptomatic control with close monitoring. Calcium channel blockers can worsen portal hypertension by causing mesenteric vasodilatation.

5.9 Portal hypertensive colopathy

Severe portal hypertension can cause lower gastrointestinal bleeding and cause anemia. Portal hypertensive colopathy has been defined endoscopically in patients with vascular ectasia, redness, and blue vein. Vascular ectasia is classified into two types: type 1, solitary vascular ectasia; and type 2, diffuse vascular ectasia. Overall portal hypertensive colopathy is found in 2/3rd of the cirrhotic patients including solitary vascular ectasia in 36%, diffuse vascular ectasia in 42%, red ness in 21% and blue vein in 12 percent [68]. Worsening of Child Pugh class and decrease in platelet count increases prevalence of portal hypertensive colopathy in patients with liver cirrhosis warranting colonoscopy to prevent lower gastrointestinal bleeding.

5.10 Cirrhotic cardiomyopathy

The diagnostic criteria of cirrhotic cardiomyopathy [69] are enumerated in **Table 5**. Decreased cardiac responsiveness (chronotropic and inotropic incompetence) through the defect in cardiac β-adrenergic receptor signaling is the main mechanism for systolic dysfunction in cirrhotic cardiomyopathy. The presence of cardiodepressant substances such as nitric oxide (NO) and carbon monoxide (CO) and endogenous cannabinoids also play role [70, 71]. Potential mechanisms for diastolic dysfunction are alteration in collagen configuration, sodium retention and activation of renin angiotensin aldosterone System (RAAS) [72].

Salt and fluid restriction, diuretics and afterload reduction are the aspects of treatment in cirrhotic cardiomyopathy. Compared with non-cirrhotics the benefit of β-blockers in cirrhotic heart failure is not clear. The use of non-selective β-blocker has been shown to reduce prolonged QT interval toward normal values in patients with cirrhosis along with some beneficial effect in improving electromechanical uncoupling [73]. Possible cure for cirrhotic cardiomyopathy is liver transplantation.

5.11 Portal biliopathy

Presence of biliary abnormalities in patients with non-cirrhotic/non-neoplastic extrahepatic portal vein obstruction (EHPVO) and portal cavernoma (PC) is called

Systolic dysfunction	Resting ejection fraction <55%
	Blunted increase in cardiac output with exercise or pharmacological stimuli
Diastolic dysfunction	Early diastolic atrial filling (E/A ratio) < 1.0 (age corrected)
	Deceleration time (DT) > 200 ms
	Prolonged isovolumetric relaxation time > 80 ms
Supportive criteria	Electrophysiological abnormalities (prolongation of QT)
	Abnormal chronotropic response
	Electromechanical uncoupling
	Enlarged left atrium
	Increased myocardial mass
	Increased brain natriuretic peptide or pro-peptide
	Increased troponin I

Table 5.
Diagnostic criteria for cirrhotic cardiomyopathy.

Stage	Portal cavernoma	Biliopathy	Liver function tests	Symptoms	Complications
Preclinic	Yes	No	Normal	No	No
Asymptomatic	Yes	Early changes	Normal or abnormal	No	No
Symptomatic	Yes	Advanced changes	Abnormal	yes	No
Complicated	Yes	Advanced changes	Abnormal	Yes	Yes

Table 6.
Characteristics of four stages in portal biliopathy natural history.

portal biliopathy. Compression of bile ducts by PC and/or to ischemic damage secondary to an altered biliary vascularization in EHPVO and PC leads to contribution of this complication.

Normally, epicholedochal venous plexus of Saint and the paracholedochal plexus of Petren, whose normal diameter does not exceed 1 mm, are responsible for the venous drainage of the biliary tree. Dilation of plexus of Saint causes fine irregularities in biliary walls while dilation of plexus of Petren causes extrinsic compression in chronic portal vein obstruction. Patients present with jaundice, cholangitis, cholecystitis, abdominal pain, and cholelithiasis. Around 5%–38% of patients develop biliary symptoms [74]. Dhiman et al. [75] identified four stages in PB progression (**Table 6**).

On the aspect of treatment, surgical porto-systemic shunt or transjugular intrahepatic porto-systemic shunt can be performed, and treatment on the biliary stenosis includes endoscopic (Endoscopic retrograde cholangiopancreatography with endoscopic sphincterotomy, balloon dilation, stone extraction, stent placement) and surgical (bilioenteric anastomosis, cholecystectomy) approaches are used for decompression of portal cavernoma.

6. Future perspectives

Besides different surgeries with portosystemic shunting, there are newer drugs developed for reduction of portal pressure. Few drugs which have been seen to be beneficial are:

6.1 Farnesoid X receptor (FXR) agonists

Obeticholic acid (OCA), a semisynthetic FXR agonist tested in preclinical models of cirrhosis has shown beneficial effects as transcriptional modulator on PH by reducing the intrahepatic vascular resistance (IHVR) [76].

6.2 Statins

Statins have antioxidative, antiproliferative and anti-inflammatory effects, and can improve endothelial dysfunction [77].

They have shown strong hepatosinusoidal protective effects in preclinical models of chronic liver diseases, ultimately leading to reduction in portal pressure [78, 79]. Simvastatin has shown beneficial effects when administered alone or combined with beta blockers [80, 81].

6.3 Anti-apoptotic drugs

Emricasan has been seen to improve portal pressure and IHVR compared with vehicle-treated rats, in addition to improved liver function and microcirculation, and finally with improved liver sinusoidal endothelial cell (LSEC) and hepatic stellate cells (HSC) phenotype and reduced inflammation [82].

6.4 Anticoagulants

Rivaroxaban, direct inhibitor of factor Xa has been shown to reduce liver microthrombosis, HSC activation and portal pressure in experimental models of cirrhosis [83].

6.5 Antidiabetic drugs

Liraglutide has shown antifibrotic effects in NASH patients, thus with high probabilities of success as a treatment for portal hypertension and chronic liver disease [84]. Metformin has shown to improve liver hemodynamic and fibrosis by a reduction in inflammation and oxidative stress [85].

6.6 Anti-inflammatory agents

Anti-inflammatory drugs such as rapamycin have reduced portal pressure in rats with Portal hypertension due to its intrahepatic and extrahepatic effects [86, 87].

6.7 Taurine

Taurine has pleiotropic effects. A small cohort of patients with clinically significant PH (HVPG >12 mmHg) has reported reduction in portal pressure [88]. Thus, consumption of low carbonated 'energy drinks' rich in taurine may have a positive impact in portal hypertension.

7. Conclusion

Portal Hypertension is responsible for many complications in liver cirrhosis. Reduction of portal pressure decreases the rate of complications in advanced liver diseases. This can improve the quality of life and increase the survival of such patients.

Conflict of interest

None.

Author details

Achyut Bikram Hamal
Nepal Police Hospital, Kathmandu, Nepal

*Address all correspondence to: abhamal@gmail.com

References

[1] Vesalius A. De Humani corporis fabrica. Basileae, 1543

[2] Glisson F. The portal circulation. In: Child G. N Engl J Med 1955; 252:837

[3] Genoveffa Balducci, Antonio V Sterpetti and Marco Ventura. A short history of portal hypertension and of its management. Journal of Gastroenterology and Hepatology 31 (2016) 541-545

[4] Dusaussey M. Etudes sur les varices de l'oesophage dans la cirrhose hepatique. These, Paris, 1877

[5] Gilbert A, Carnot P. Les fonctions hepatiques. Paris, 1902

[6] Davidson CS, Gibbons TB, Faloon WW. Systemic and portal venous pressures in cirrhosis of the liver. J Lab Clin Med 1950; 35:181

[7] Thompson WP, Caughley GL, Whipple AO et al. Splein vein pressure in congestive splenomegaly. J. Clin. Invest. 1937; 16: 571-576.

[8] Lebon J, Fabregoule M, Eisenbeth H et al. Splenoportographie transperietale. Alg Med 1953; 57: 105-110.

[9] Abraldes JG, Sarlieve P, Tandon P. Measurement of portal pressure. Clinics in liver disease. 2014 Nov 1;18(4):779-792.

[10] John C. Hoefs, et al. Diagnosis and hemodynamic assessment of portal hypertension. Surgical Clinics of North America-Vol. 70, No.2, April 1990

[11] Bosch J, Abraldes JG, Berzigotti A, et al. The clinical use of HVPG measurements in chronic liver disease. Nat Rev Gastroenterol Hepatol 2009;6: 576-582.

[12] Groszmann RJ, Glickman M, Blei AT, et al. Wedged and free hepatic venous pressure measured with a balloon catheter. Gastroenterology 1979;76(2):253-258.

[13] La Mura V, Abraldes JG, Berzigotti A, et al. Right atrial pressure is not adequate to calculate portal pressure gradient in cirrhosis: a clinical-hemodynamic correlation study. Hepatology 2010; 51(6):2108-2116.

[14] Abraldes JG, Araujo IK, Turon F, et al. Diagnosing and monitoring cirrhosis: liver biopsy, hepatic venous pressure gradient and elastography. Gastroenterol Hepatol 2012;35(7):488-495.

[15] Kumar M, Kumar A, Hissar S et al. Hepatic venous pressure gradient as a predictor of ¢ brosis in chronic liver disease because of hepatitis B virus. Liver Int 2008; 28: 690-698.

[16] Blasco A, Forns X, Carrion JA et al. Hepatic venous pressure gradient identifies patients at risk of severe hepatitis C recurrence after liver transplantation. Hepatology 2006; 43: 492-499.

[17] Garcia-Tsao G, Groszmann RJ, Fisher RL et al. Portal pressure, presence of gastroesophageal varices and variceal bleeding. Hepatology 1985; 5: 419-424.

[18] Groszmann RJ, Garcia-Tsao G, Bosch J et al. Beta-blockers to prevent gastroesophageal varices in patients with cirrhosis. N Engl J Med 2005; 353:2254-2261.

[19] Ripoll C, Groszmann R, Garcia-Tsao G et al. Hepatic venous pressure gradient predicts clinical decompensation in patients with compensated cirrhosis. Gastroenterology 2007; 133:481-488.

[20] Ripoll C, Groszmann RJ, Garcia-Tsao G et al. Hepatic venous pressure gradient predicts development of hepatocellular carcinoma independently

of severity of cirrhosis. J Hepatol 2009; 50: 923-928.

[21] Berzigotti A, Reig M, Abraldes JG et al. Portal hypertension and the outcome of surgery for hepatocellular carcinoma in compensated cirrhosis: a systematic review and meta-analysis. Hepatology 2015; 61: 526-536

[22] Habib A, Sanyal AJ. Acute variceal hemorrhage. Gastrointest Endosc Clin N Am 2007; 17:223-252, v.

[23] De Franchis R, Dell'Era A, Iannuzzi F. Diagnosis and treatment of portal hypertension. Dig Liver Dis. 2004; 36:787-798.

[24] Silva-Junior G, Baiges A, Turon F et al. The prognostic value of hepatic venous pressure gradient in patients with cirrhosis is highly dependent on the accuracy of the technique. Hepatology 2015; 62:1584-1592.

[25] Abraldes JG, Villanueva C, Banares R ~ et al. Hepatic venous pressure gradient and prognosis in patients with acute variceal bleeding treated with pharmacologic and endoscopic therapy. J Hepatol 2008;48: 229-236.

[26] Rincon D, Lo Iacono O, Ripoll C et al. Prognostic value of hepatic venous pressure gradient for in-hospital mortality of patients with severe acute alcoholic hepatitis. Aliment Pharmacol Ther 2007; 25:841-848.

[27] Serste T, Bourgeois N, Lebrec D, Evrard S, Devière J, Le Moine O. Relationship between the degree of portal hypertension and the onset of spontaneous bacterial peritonitis in patients with cirrhosis. Acta gastro-enterologica Belgica. 2006;69(4):355.

[28] Berzigotti A, Seijo S, Reverter E, Bosch J, Bosch, Groszmann; Portal Hypertension Collaborative Group, Casado, García-Pagán, Fernández, Roskams. Assessing portal hypertension in liver diseases. Expert review of gastroenterology & hepatology. 2013 Feb 1;7(2):141-155.

[29] Groszmann RJ, Wongcharatrawee S. The hepatic venous pressure gradient: anything worth doing should be done right. Hepatology. 2004 Feb;39(2): 280-283.

[30] Bosch J, Navasa M, Garcia-Pagan JC, Delacy AM, Rodes J: Portal hypertension. Med Clin North Am 1989; 73:931-953.

[31] Thompson R, Taylor M, McKie L, Diamond T. Sinistral Portal Hyper-tension. Ulster Med J. 2006; 75 (3) 175-177.

[32] Singhal D, Kakodkar R, Soin A, Gupta S, Nundy S. Sinistral Portal Hypertension. A Case Report. JOP. 2006; 7(6):670-667.

[33] Koklu S, Coban S, Yuksel O, Arhan M. Left-Sided Portal Hypertension. Dig Dis Sci. 2007; 52:1141-1149

[34] Li ZS, Tang CW, Qian JM, Yuan YZ, Wang XP. Practice guidance for diagnosis and treatment of pancreatitis-related splanchnic vein thrombosis (Shenyang, 2020). Journal of Digestive Diseases. 2020 Nov 20.

[35] Adams DB, Mauterer DJ, Vujic IJ, Anderson MD. Preoperative control of splenic artery inflow in patients with splenic venous occlusion. South Med J. 1990; 83:1021-1024.

[36] Habib A, Sanyal AJ. Acute variceal hemorrhage. Gastrointest Endosc Clin N Am 2007; 17:223-252, v.

[37] Zaman A. Current Management of Esophageal Varices. Curr Treat Options Gastroenterol 2003; 6:499-507

[38] Carbonell N, Pauwels A, Serfaty L, Fourdan O, Lévy VG, Poupon R.et al. Improved survival after variceal bleeding in patients with cirrhosis over

the past two decades. Hepatology2004; 40:652-659.

[39] Castaneda B, Debernardi-Venon W, Bandi JC Andreu V, Pérez-del-Pulgar S, Moitinho E, Pizcueta P, Bosch J.et al. The role of portal pressure in the severity of bleeding in portal hypertensive rats. Hepatology2000; 31:581-586

[40] Russo MW. Variceal Bleeding. Curr Treat Options Gastroenterol. 2002; 5:471-477.

[41] Bernard B, Lebrec D, Mathurin P, Opolon P, Poynard T. Beta-adrenergic antagonists in the prevention of gastro-intestinal rebleeding in patients with cirrhosis: a meta-analysis. Hepatology 1997; 25:63-70.

[42] De Franchis R. Evolving consensus in portal hypertension. Report of the Baveno IV consensus workshop on methodology of diagnosis and therapy in portal hypertension. J Hepatol 2005; 43:167-176

[43] Bosch J, Garcia-Pagan JC. Prevention of variceal rebleeding. Lancet 2003; 361:952-954.

[44] Hamal AB, KC S, Thapa P, Sharma D, Karki N, et al. Carvedilol Versus Propranolol for Secondary Prophylaxis of Variceal Hemorrhage in Patients with Liver Cirrhosis. Adv Res Gastroentero Hepatol, 2020; 15(4): 555920.

[45] Kamath PS, Shah VH: Portal Hypertension and Bleeding Esophageal Varices. Zakim and Boyer's Hepatology: A Textbook of Liver Disease (6th ed). In Boyer TD, Manns MP, Sanyal AJ (ed): Elsevier Saunders, Philadelphia; 2012. 296-326.

[46] Feldman M, Lee EL: Pathophysiology, Diagnosis, Management. Sleisenger and Fordtran's Gastrointestinal and Liver Disease (10th ed). In: Feldman M, Friedman LS, Brandt LJ (ed): Elsevier Saunders, Philadelphia; 2010. 868-883

[47] Vigneri S, Termini R, Piraino A, Scialabba A, Pisciotta G, Fontana N: The stomach in liver cirrhosis. Endoscopic, morphological, and clinical correlations. Gastroenterology. 1991,101:472-478.

[48] McCormack TT, Sims J, Eyre-Brook I, Kennedy H, Goepel J, Johnson AG, Triger DR: Gastric lesions in portal hypertension: inflammatory gastritis or congestive gastropathy? Gut. 1985,26:1226-1232.

[49] Tiwari P S, Kc S, Sharma D, et al. (August 21, 2019) Prevalence of Portal Hypertensive Gastropathy in Chronic Liver Disease and Correlation with the Severity of Liver disease. Cureus 11(8): e5454.

[50] Gjeorgjievski M, Cappell MS: Portal hypertensive gastropathy: a systematic review of the pathophysiology, clinical presentation, natural history and therapy. World J Hepatol. 2016, 8:231-262.

[51] Primignani M, Carpinelli L, Preatoni P, Battaglia G, Carta A, Prada A, Cestari R, Angeli P, Gatta A, Rossi A, Spinzi G. Natural history of portal hypertensive gastropathy in patients with liver cirrhosis. Gastroenterology. 2000 Jul 1; 119(1): 181-187.

[52] Bates JA. Abdominal Ultrasound. 2nd ed. Edinburgh: Churchill Livingstone; 2004. p. 97-107.

[53] Moore KP, Wong F, Gines P, Bernardi M, Ochs A, Salerno F, Angeli P, Porayko M, Moreau R, Garcia-Tsao G, Jimenez W. The management of ascites in cirrhosis: report on the consensus conference of the International Ascites Club. Hepatology. 2003 Jul 1;38(1):258-266.

[54] Ding X, Yu Y, Chen M, Wang C, Kang Y, Lou J. Causative agents and outcome of spontaneous bacterial peritonitis in cirrhotic patients: community-acquired versus nosocomial

infections. BMC infectious diseases. 2019 Dec 1; 19(1):463.

[55] Acharya SK. Difficult to treat spontaneous bacterial peritonitis. Tropical Gastroenterology. 2013 May 18;34(1):7-13.

[56] Elsadek HM, Elhawari SA, Mokhtar A. A novel serum index for accurate diagnosis of spontaneous bacterial peritonitis in cirrhotic patients without other infections. Egyptian Liver Journal. 2020 Dec; 10(1):1-8.

[57] Enomoto H, Inoue SI, Matsuhisa A, Nishiguchi S. Diagnosis of spontaneous bacterial peritonitis and an in situ hybridization approach to detect an "unidentified" pathogen. International journal of hepatology. 2014 Jan 1; 2014.

[58] Epstein M. Hepatorenal syndrome: emerging perspectives of pathophysiology and therapy. J Am Soc Nephrol JASN. 1994 Apr;4(10):1735-1753

[59] Low G, Alexander GJM, Lomas DJ. Hepatorenal Syndrome: Aetiology, Diagnosis, and Treatment [Internet]. Gastroenterology Research and Practice. 2015.

[60] Angeli P et al. News in pathophysiology, definition and classification of hepatorenal syndrome: A step beyond the International Club of Ascites (ICA) consensus document. J Hepatol (2019).

[61] Garbuzenko DV, Arefyev NO. Hepatic hydrothorax: An update and review of the literature. World J Hepatol 2017; 9(31): 1197-1204

[62] Lazaridis KN, Frank JW, Krowka MJ, Kamath PS. Hepatic hydrothorax: pathogenesis, diagnosis, and manageent. Am J Med 1999; 107: 262-267.

[63] Huang PM, Chang YL, Yang CY, Lee YC. The morphology of diaphragmatic defects in hepatic hydrothorax: thoracoscopic finding. J Thorac Cardiovasc Surg 2005; 130: 141-145.

[64] The European Association for the Study of the Liver. EASL Clinical Practice Guidelines for the management of patients with decompensated cirrhosis. J Hepatol (2018), https://doi.org/10.1016/j.jhep.2018.03.024.

[65] De BK, Dutta D, Pal SK, Gangopadhyay S, Das Baksi S, Pani A. The role of garlic in hepatopulmonary syndrome: a randomized controlled trial. Can J Gastroenterol 2010; 24:183-188.

[66] Porres-Aguilar M, Gallegos-Orozco JF, Garcia H, Aguirre J, Macias-Rodriguez RU, Torre-Delgadillo A. Pulmonary vascular complications in portal hypertension and liver disease: a concise review. Rev Gastroenterol Mex. 2013;78(1):35-44. doi: 10.1016/j.rgmx.2012.10.004.

[67] Hadengue A, Benhayoun MK, Lebrec D, Benhamou JP. Pulmonary hypertension complicating portal hypertension: prevalence and relation to splanchnic hemodynamics. Gastroenterology. 1991 Feb 1; 100(2): 520-528.

[68] Ito K, Shiraki K, Sakai T, Yoshimura H, Nakano T. Portal hypertensive colopathy in patients with liver cirrhosis. World Journal of Gastroenterology: WJG. 2005 May 28; 11(20):3127.

[69] Wiese S, Hove JD, Bendtsen F, Møller S. Cirrhotic cardiomyopathy: pathogenesis and clinical relevance. Nature reviews Gastroenterology & hepatology. 2014 Mar;11(3):177.

[70] Baldassarre M, Giannone FA, Napoli L, Tovoli A, Ricci CS, Tufoni M, et al. The endocannabinoid system in advanced liver cirrhosis: pathophysiological implication and future perspectives. Liver Int. 2013;33: 1298-1308.

[71] Van Obbergh L, Vallieres Y, Blaise G. Cardiac modifications occurring in the ascitic rat with biliary cirrhosis are nitric oxide related. J Hepatol. 1996;24: 747-752.

[72] Wong F. Cirrhotic cardiomyopathy. Hepatol Int. 2009; 3:294-304.

[73] Henriksen JH, Bendtsen F, Hansen EF, Moller S. Acute non-selective beta-adrenergic blockade reduces prolonged frequency-adjusted Q-T interval (QTc) in patients with cirrhosis. J Hepatol. 2004; 40:239-246.

[74] Franceschet I, Zanetto A, Ferrarese A, Burra P, Senzolo M. Therapeutic approaches for portal biliopathy: A systematic review. World J Gastroenterol. 2016 Dec 7; 22(45):9909-9920.

[75] Dhiman RK, Saraswat VA, Valla DC, Chawla Y, Behera A, Varma V, Agarwal S, Duseja A, Puri P, Kalra N, et al. Portal cavernoma cholangiopathy: consensus statement of a working party of the Indian national association for study of the liver. J Clin Exp Hepatol. 2014;4: S2–S14.

[76] Verbeke L, Farre R, Trebicka J, Komuta M, Roskams T, Klein S, Elst IV, Windmolders P, Vanuytsel T, Nevens F, Laleman W. Obeticholic acid, a farnesoid X receptor agonist, improves portal hypertension by two distinct pathways in cirrhotic rats. Hepatology. 2014 Jun; 59(6):2286-2298.

[77] Pose E, Trebicka J, Mookerjee RP, Angeli P, Ginès P. Statins: old drugs as new therapy for liver diseases? Journal of hepatology. 2019 Jan 1;70(1):194-202.

[78] Trebicka J, Hennenberg M, Laleman W, et al. Atorvastatin lowers portal pressure in cirrhotic rats by inhibition of RhoA/Rho-kinase and activation of endothelial nitric oxide synthase. Hepatology 2007; 46: 242-253.

[79] Abraldes JG, Rodríguez-Vilarrupla A, Graupera M, et al. Simvastatin treatment improves liver sinusoidal endothelial dysfunction in CCl4 cirrhotic rats. J Hepatol 2007; 46: 1040-1046.

[80] Pollo-Flores P, Soldan M, Santos UC, et al. Three months of simvastatin therapy vs. placebo for severe portal hypertension in cirrhosis: a randomized controlled trial. Dig Liver Dis 2015; 47: 957-963.

[81] Abraldes JG, Villanueva C, Aracil C, et al. Addition of simvastatin to standard therapy for the prevention of variceal rebleeding does not reduce rebleeding but increases survival in patients with cirrhosis. Gastroenterology 2016; 150: 1160-1170.e3

[82] Gracia-Sancho J, Contreras PC, Vila S, et al. The pan caspase inhibitor emricasan improves the hepatic microcirculatory dysfunction of CCl4-cirrhotic rats leading to portal hypertension amelioration and cirrhosis regression. Hepatology 2016; 64: 811-1050.

[83] Vilaseca M, García-Calderó H, Lafoz E, et al. The anticoagulant rivaroxaban lowers portal hypertension in cirrhotic rats mainly by deactivating hepatic stellate cells. Hepatology 2017; 65: 2031-2044.

[84] Armstrong MJ, Gaunt P, Aithal GP, et al. Liraglutide safety and efficacy in patients with non-alcoholic steatohepatitis (LEAN): a multicentre, double-blind, randomised, placebo-controlled phase 2 study. Lancet 2016; 387: 679-690.

[85] Tripathi DM, Erice E, Lafoz E, et al. Metformin reduces hepatic resistance and portal pressure in cirrhotic rats. Am J Physiol Gastrointest Liver Physiol 2015; 309: G301–G309.

[86] Wang W, Yan J, Wang H, et al. Rapamycin ameliorates inflammation and fibrosis in the early phase of

cirrhotic portal hypertension in rats through inhibition of mTORC1 but not mTORC2. PLoS One 2014; 9: e83908.

[87] Mejias M, Garcia-Pras E, Gallego J, et al. Relevance of the mTOR signaling pathway in the pathophysiology of splenomegaly in rats with chronic portal hypertension. J Hepatol 2010; 52: 529-539.

[88] Schwarzer R, Kivaranovic D, Mandorfer M, Paternostro R, Wolrab D, Heinisch B, Reiberger T, Ferlitsch M, Gerner C, Trauner M, Peck-Radosavljevic M. Randomised clinical study: the effects of oral taurine 6 g/day vs placebo on portal hypertension. Alimentary pharmacology & therapeutics. 2018 Jan; 47(1):86-94.

Chapter 2

Pediatric Portal Hypertension

Reda A. Zbaida

Abstract

Portal hypertension is increased intravascular pressure of the portal vein. The prevalence of causes in children is different from adults ones. The commonest cause of pediatric portal hypertension is the extra-hepatic portal hypertension, comparing with an adult where liver cirrhosis is the comments cause. Also, taking into consideration, the fundamental physiological differences between the two age groups. These elements are making the attempt to extrapolate the adult guidelines to the pediatric age group unpractical. On the other hand, the limitation of well-designed studies in the pediatric age group makes reaching a consensus about the safety and efficiency of primary prophylaxis of variceal bleeding difficult. In contrast, there were enough data to recommend the secondary prophylaxis of variceal bleeding and the safety and efficiency of Meso-Rex shunt for portal hypertension have been confirmed. These indicate the necessity of further studies to reach a complete algorithm of guidelines for pediatric portal hypertension.

Keywords: portal hypertension, children, esophageal varices, variceal bleeding, selective shunts, non-selective shunts

1. Introduction

The portal hypertension is caused by an increased resistance to venous flow in portal vein. Which leads to an increase to pressure in the portal circulation. It is a result of chronic liver disease, obstruction of portal vein, or portosystemic shunt, which leads to hyperdynamic circulation.

The normal hepatic venous pressure gradient (HVPG) correlates with normal portal pressure which is 1–4 mm Hg. A pressure gradient of more than 10 mm Hg links to esophageal varices. The pressure 12 mm Hg predicts the risk of active bleeding. [1]

The most common complication of pediatric portal hypertension is acute variceal bleeding. The grading system of the Japanese Research Society for Portal Hypertension of esophageal varices is as follows: grade 1: flattened by insufflation, grade 2: not flattened by insufflation but is not circumferential, grade 3: not flattened and is circumferential. [2]

2. Embryology

The three main venous embryo systems will be recognizable by the end of the 3rd week of gestation.

They include (1) the 2 cardinal veins which drain the embryo blood (intra-embryonic system). To the sinus venosus (primitive atrium). The other two are extraembryonic systems, one of them transports the blood from the yolk sac to the heart (sinus venosus) which is called (2) the vitelline veins (two pairs). Finally, (3) the 2 umbilical veins transport the oxygenated blood from the placenta to the embryo's heart. [3]

The hepatic bud starts branching off from the caudal end of the foregut, which expands into the transversum septum (Mesenchymal tissue in the pericardiac area). The cephalic part of the hepatic bud will eventually form the liver. And the caudal part will form the biliary tree and the gall bladder. During liver development, the primitive liver tissue in the transversum septum is in close contact with the two extraembryonic venous systems (**Figure 1**).

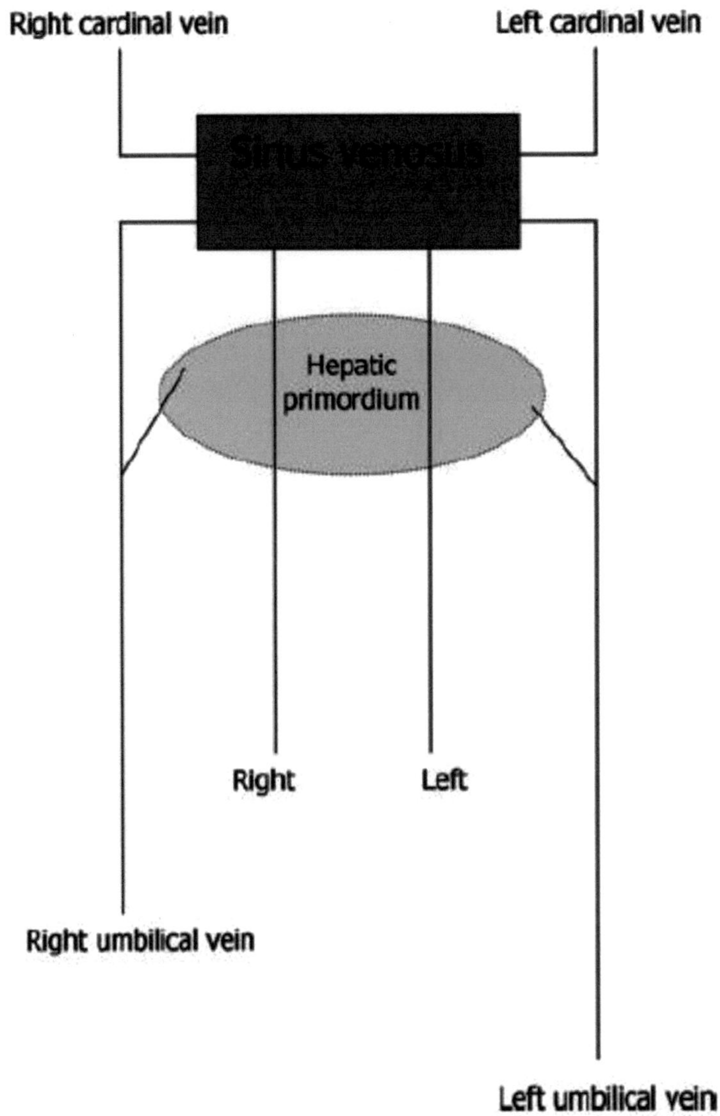

Figure 1.
Schematic drawing represents the relation between the primitive hepatic bud and the major fetal venous systems. (Courtesy of Collardeau-Frachon and Scoazec et al. [4]. All the rights reserved).

The portal circulation of the liver develops between the 4th and 6th weeks, which is the result of a complex interaction between a primitive liver and a pair of vitelline veins and umbilical veins.

Initially, the vitelline veins form 4 sites of anastomoses between each other in their way to the sinus venosus, which are the caudal-ventral anastomosis, middle dorsal (they named according to their relation to the foregut), subhepatic, and finally the subdiaphragmatic anastomosis.

A net of smaller anastomoses between the right and the left vitelline veins extend in the area between the subdiaphragmatic and the subhepatic anastomoses in the same site where the hepatic bud will proliferate and develop to form the liver (the caudal part of the septum transversum). Synchronously, the umbilical veins in their way to the sinus venosus each vein are divided into 2 branches. One runs in parallel to the primitive liver and the other one ends in the liver parenchyma. The right umbilical vein and its branches atrophy in the 4th week. Also, the direct branch to the sinus venosus disappears in the same period. But the left branch of the umbilical vein to the liver parenchyma persists. It increases in size gradually inside liver parenchyma till communicates with the left end of the subhepatic anastomosis of the vitelline veins. That is known as a portal sinus. So, all the oxygenated blood is conveyed to the liver via the left umbilical vein. Due to massive blood influx to the liver, one of the anastomosing veins between the subhepatic and subdiaphragmatic anastomoses increases in size tremendously (Ductus venosus) to accommodate the oxygenated blood from the portal sinus to sinus venosus via a subdiaphragmatic anastomosis. [4]

The future portal vein is formed of the inferior section of the left vitelline vein, middle dorsal anastomosis, and the superior section of the right vitelline vein. By end of this process in the 6th week, the S-shape portal vein starts to appear. By this, the definitive fetal portal circulation is formed. [4]

The next major event happens at birth when the umbilical blood flow ceases. Subsequently, intravascular pressure in the umbilical vein and the ductus venosus drop and obliterating of these veins start within minutes after birth, which usually takes 15–20 days for complete closure. [3]

3. Anatomy and collateral circulation

The portal vein is formed by the union of the superior mesenteric and the splenic veins behind the neck of the pancreas. It passes behind the first part of the duodenum, then it runs in the free edge of the lesser momentum posterior to the common bile duct (on the right side) and hepatic artery proper (on the left side) up to the porta hepatis where it divides into right and the left portal veins. Both main branches continue breaking down up to the sinusoids.

There is a specific pattern of the breakdown of the portal vein, the biliary duct, and hepatic arteries within the liver parenchyma, which does not correlate with the liver surface anatomy.

The Cantlie's line extends from the inferior vena cava to the fundus of the gall bladder, which divides the liver into right and left lobes. Cantlie's line represents the true surgical division of the liver into right and left lobes. [5]

The description of further portal triad breakdowns and its correlation with hepatic veins is delineated by a French surgeon and anatomist "Claude Couinaud", depending on his framework that every half further divides into sectors, and a hepatic sector according to Couinaud system (**Figure 2**) is a region bounded by 2 hepatic veins or a hepatic vein and the hepatic edge. And the segment in the region

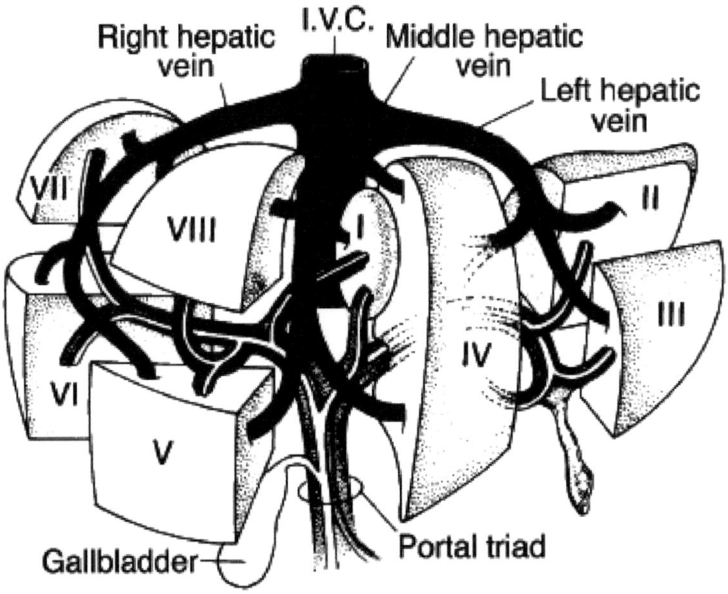

Figure 2.
Drawing represents the Couinaud system and the relation of left portal vein to ligamentous teres in the umbilical fissure. (Courtesy of John E. Skandalakis et al. [6], All rights reserved).

of the liver that has an independent portal triad (separate branches from the portal vein, the hepatic artery, and the biliary duct) supplies it. These anatomical facts guide the hepatobiliary surgeons to execute the hepatectomy (right or left) and segmentectomy precisely. [7]

The location of the Rex recess has an important surgical application in pediatric portal hypertension. That is where a branch from the left portal branch lies in the porto-umbilical fissure between the left lateral sector (segments II, III) and the left medial sector (segment IV). In intrauterine life, the left portal branch in the recess of Rex was communicating with the left umbilical vein. The fibrous remnant of the left umbilical postnatally known as ligamentous teres can be used as a reliable anatomical landmark for the recess of the Rex, which is surgically accessible and connecting it to the mesenteric vessel (superior mesenteric vein) via graft to bypass the portal occlusion and avoid the cavernoma, which is a net of collaterals formed after the portal obstruction in the area of porta hepatis. A portal vein occlusion is the commonest cause of portal hypertension in the pediatric age group.

Another important anatomical aspect of portal hypertension is the collateral anastomoses [8] between the portal and systemic circulations. Under normal circumstances, the mesenteric vein returns to the liver via the portal vein, then to the inferior vena cava (systemic circulation) via the hepatic veins to reach finally, the right atrium of the heart. This normal pathway would be interrupted in portal hypertension where the resistance to blood flow in the portal circulation is increased. This forces the blood to use the porto-systemic anastomoses as alternative pathways to reach the systemic circulation, which are negligible in normal situations. But in portal hypertension, these anastomoses increase in size with the increased potentiality of hemorrhage (ex: esophageal varices).

These anastomoses are as follows:

- The esophageal branches of the left gastric vein (a tributary of the portal circulation) anastomose with esophageal branches of hemiazygos vein (systemic circulation).

- The anastomosis between the superior rectal vein (portal circulation) with the middle and inferior rectal veins (systemic circulation) in the anal canal.
- Paraumbilical anastomoses (caput medusa) are the communication between tributaries of portal vein which run in the falciform with the superficial veins of the anterior abdominal wall.
- The communications between veins of ascending colon, descending colon, and duodenum (portal circulation) with the left renal vein (systemic circulation).
- The veins of Retzius connect retroperitoneally between tributaries of inferior vena cava and tributaries of the superior and inferior mesenteric veins.
- The accessory portal system of sappey is a set of diaphragmatic veins connecting the portal system to the systemic system.

4. Causes

The spectrum of causes is arranged in the pre-hepatic, the hepatic, and the post-hepatic lesions.

- *Pre-hepatic lesions:* Extra-hepatic portal vein obstruction is the commonest cause of portal hypertension. The underlying cause of portal thrombosis is unidentifiable in most cases. [9] But it links to the predisposing factors. They are an injury to the portal vein in the cannulation of the umbilical vein, dehydration, abdominal sepsis, omphalitis, and hypercoagulable state. Another factor is the extra-mural compression like enlarged lymph node due to inflammation or malignancy. [10]

  The portosystemic shunt is another cause of portal hypertension which can be surgical or iatrogenic cause or congenital shunts. Lautz et al. proposed a classification for congenital portosystemic shunts which divide them into 2 types. Type I with no intrahepatic portal venous flow. Type II with some intrahepatic portal venous flow. [11]

- *Hepatic lesions:* Hepatic cellular injury of any cause (e.g. Biliary atresia, Schistosomiasis) stimulates collagen deposition via activated stellate cells, which leads to an increase resistance to venous outflow. [12]
- *Post-hepatic lesions:* They include the hepatic veno-occlusive disease. [13] Busulfan containing regimes use for a bone marrow ablation in the bone marrow transplant considered are risk factors for hepatic veno-occlusive disease, because of hepatic and endothelial cellular injuries, which cause hepatic venules obstruction leading to venous congestion and eventually, to portal hypertension. Budd-Chiari syndrome is another cause of post-hepatic obstruction. Although it is uncommon in the pediatric age group, Budd-Chiari syndrome does occur in children. The level of obstruction can be at any level from the hepatic veins up to the level of the aortocaval junction. The most underlying cause of Budd-Chiari syndrome in children is the hypercoagulable state (Protein C, S deficiency, antithrombin III deficiency). [14]

5. Clinical presentations

How the pediatric patient with portal hypertension is presented depends on 2 essential factors: (1) the site of the obstruction (2) whether the patient has liver cirrhosis or not.

- *Upper GI bleeding:* It is a frightening and common presenting symptom of portal hypertension in the pediatric age group. About 70% of the extra-hepatic portal hypertension cases present with upper GI bleeding, which is the common cause of pediatric portal hypertension presented. [10] But since the liver parenchyma and functions are preserved for decades in the extra-hepatic portal hypertension at the time of the presentation almost all the patients have a normal liver function. For this reason, most of these patients recovered without serious complications with a low mortality rate. This is true for all patients with compensated liver function presented with upper GI bleeding. Unfortunately, this is not the case for patients with decompensated liver disease (cirrhosis). Mathieu Duche et al. in their study reported that 1/5 of patients with cirrhosis developed life-threatening complications after upper GI bleeds. [15]

- *Portal hypertensive gastropathy:* It is gastric lesions related to portal hypertensive disease. It ranges from erythema to diffuse gastritis. It is an occasional cause of upper GI bleeding. But it most commonly causes iron deficiency anemia due to chronic blood loss, which also may manifest as melena. [16]

- *Splenomegaly and hypersplenism:* Splenomegaly alone could be the presenting symptom in the extra-hepatic portal hypertension, in this scenario usually there are no other hepatic signs and symptoms, which necessitates excluding hematologic causes. If the patient has cirrhosis, the signs, and symptoms of liver disease (e.g. spider naevi, jaundice, ascites) will be presented with *splenomegaly*. *Splenomegaly* imposes a significant risk in adolescent patients due to the type of sports and activities involved in this age group. It may lead to a spleen rupture and catastrophic bleeding. Splenectomy may be the only option in these patients, who do not complaint about avoiding contact sports. Also, these patients may develop hypersplenism (*splenomegaly,* with thrombocytopenia and leukopenia). [17] Although the *hepatomegaly* is not common in pediatric portal hypertension. But it could be associated with Budd-Chiari syndrome and congenital hepatic fibrosis. [14, 18]

- *Encephalopathy:* It is a known complication of liver cirrhosis. But it can be associated with normal liver function in the extra-hepatic portal hypertension patients caused by port-systemic shunts, whether it is congenital or systemic shunts. It could be manifested as learning difficulties and behavior abnormalities. [19]

- *Pulmonary related disorders: Pulmonary hypertension* is associated with portal hypertension with or without liver disease. [20] It is caused by increased vascular resistance due to pulmonary vasoconstriction as a result of shunting vasoactive substance to the systemic circulation whether is due to prehepatic shunting or inability of the liver to process the proteins (liver cirrhosis). And the *hepatopulmonary syndrome* is the contrast to *pulmonary hypertension,* which present with dyspnea and hypoxia resulting from pulmonary arteriovenous shunting and partial oxygenation of the blood due to massive capillary dilation as a response to vasodilators proteins bypassed to the systemic circulation. [21]

Patients with portal hypertension may present with signs of liver disease if the underlying cause of portal hypertension is the damage of liver parenchyma. For example, *Ascites* develops due to 2 important factors: (1) protein synthesis failure in the liver which impairs the intravascular oncotic pressure (2) dilated abdominal vascular capillaries and lymphatic microcirculation as a result of the increased portal hydrostatic pressure. [22] *Jaundice* is another sign of decompensated liver function. It happens due to the inability of the liver to process the bilirubin as one product of hemoglobin breakdown. [23]

6. Work up

- *Blood investigation:*

- *Complete blood count (CBC):* It is useful to identify the presence of and type of anemia. Also, it is essential in the management of acute variceal bleeding. The presence of thrombocytopenia and leukopenia in portal hypertension investigation usually indicate hypersplenism.

- *Liver function test:* It assesses the functionality of the liver. That will help to point toward the underlying cause of portal hypertension with help of other investigation modalities (see later). Low protein level (albumin) and prolonged coagulation profile indicate the impaired synthetic ability of the liver. The increased bilirubin level and hepatic enzymes indicate hepatocellular damage.

- *Renal function test:* It assesses dehydration especially in acute variceal bleeding, and impaired renal function test associated with liver diseases, like congenital hepatic fibrosis which linked to polycystic kidney disease.

Other investigations are requested according to the clinical status of the patients. Blood glucose will be low in decompensated liver cirrhosis and it is low in glycogen storage disease. Also, the ammonia level is indicated to confirm the diagnosis of encephalopathy. The coagulation screen in liver cirrhosis is prolonged. But in the extra-hepatic portal thrombosis, the coagulation profile shows secondary hypercoagulable abnormalities. [24] It will be reversed after the obstruction is overcomed.

- *Endoscopy:* It is an essential tool in portal hypertension management. It confirms the presence of varices in the esophagus and the stomach and identifies the cause of the upper GI bleeding whether from varices or other origins like hemorrhagic gastritis or Mallory-Weiss syndrome. Also, in cases of acute upper GI bleeding are not responsive to medical management, endoscopy offers an important therapeutic option to control the variceal bleeding whether via variceal banding or sclerotherapy. [25]

- *Radiological modalities:* The first radiological modality in use as part of the diagnosis armamentarium is an abdominal ultrasound with Doppler. It provides a lot of important and useful information, which include the size, echogenicity of the liver, and presence of the cysts or nodules. It also delineates the status of the intra and extra biliary tree, the patency of the portal vein, and the presence of the cavernoma in the porta hepatis. The size and echogenicity of the spleen are demonstrated in the abdominal ultrasound. And by assessing the vascularity of the abdomen it can provide valuable information for the surgical team such as the patency of the superior mesenteric, renal, and splenic veins. The neck Doppler ultrasound plays an important role in planning for surgical intervention, by confirming the patency of Jugular veins. This allows using one of them as an autologous graft provided both veins are patent. [26] Furthermore, the distance between the veins can assess the possibility of shunting between them like the distance between the renal and the spleen veins to assess the possibility of the splenorenal shunting. It may also pick up the portosystemic shunting. But the computed tomography angiography and magnetic resonance angiography are more accurate to pick up such anomalies. The later radiological modalities are usually the second step in the work up to delineate the anatomy more accurately. Invasive radiological investigations are required in specific cases. For example, the wedged hepatic venography is required in the congenital porto-systemic shunts [27] and to check the patency of the left portal vein tributary in the Rex recess to assess the possibility of Rex shunt.

7. Management of acute variceal bleeding

The upper GI bleeding can be the first presenting symptom of pediatric portal hypertension, especially when the extra-hepatic portal vein thrombosis is the underlying cause of portal hypertension. The mortality risk from the first variceal bleeding is less than 1% in pediatric portal hypertension. [28] This is due to 2 facts. First, portal hypertension in children develops early in course of the pathology, which leads subsequently to early variceal formation in children who have well-compensated liver function. Thus, the ability of the children's recover is better comparing with adults (adult mortality rate ranging from 7 to 15%). Secondly, improved medical management reduce the mortality rate in all age groups. [12]

The management of acute variceal bleeding should start with securing the airway. Insertion 2 large cannulas withdraw the blood simultaneously for urgent investigations, which should include complete blood count, blood crossmatch, urea and electrolytes, liver function test, and blood clotting profile. The other blood tests as the medical situation are mandatory. [12]

The volume replacement should start as soon as possible with crystalloids and packed red blood cells aiming to maintain the hemoglobin at or above 7 g/dL. [25] This strategy prevents tissue hypoxia which reduces lactic acid accumulation in the tissues and blood. Therefore, blood acidosis becomes less likely. Eventually, the impairment of clotting factors (proteins) function also becomes less likely. This strategy hinders the slipping towards deleterious complications of disseminated intravascular coagulopathy. The insertion of the nasogastric tube is also beneficial in observing the continuity of the bleeding and evacuating the blood of the stomach. Evacuation of the blood from the stomach has significant importance in cirrhotic patients to prevent encephalopathy. The octreotide is a synthetic analogue of somatostatin, which reduces the portal venous inflow by constriction of the splanchnic arterioles via a direct effect on the arteriole smooth muscles. It is started as a bolus dose (1 mcg/kg) followed by infusion (1 mcg/kg/H) usually for 4–5 days, which is often followed endoscopy after controlling the bleeding. [29] The only accepted situations to use endoscopic sclerotherapy in children should be acute bleeding not responding to the medical management with technical difficulty to apply band and infant's cases where there is no banding device available for them. There is a randomized trial showing the administration of erythromycin intravenously by 30 minutes before the endoscopy improves visibility and reduces the time of the procedure. [30] In a situation where medical management (including the endoscopy) fails to stop the bleeding, urgent shunt surgery or trans-jugular intrahepatic portosystemic shunt (TIPS) should be performed. The optimal environment for the management of these patients is the intensive care unit, where all the vital signs are monitored closely.

8. Primary prophylaxis

The primary prophylaxis aims to prevent the first variceal bleeding. The efficiency of the primary prophylaxis is well established in adult by screening the portal hypertension patients and identify the high-risk elements for variceal bleeding like the large size of varices (Grade 2,3), presence of the red wale on varices' surface, and the severity of the liver disease. [31] Using the endoscopic banding and/or non-selective beta-blockers which act by decreasing the portal pressure via un-opposed action of alfa-receptor on the splanchnic arterioles and decreasing the cardiac output. Sclerotherapy is not recommended for primary prophylaxis because of increased mortality in one randomized study which is forced the discontinuity of this study. [32] Regarding the children, there is no consensus about the primary prophylaxis in the pediatric age group because there is no substantial data to decide which patients need screening and what are the predictive factors for variceal presence. [28] Some studies indicate that the presence of varices in children should be related to low albumin levels, increased size of the spleen, and thrombocytopenia. But there is a need for larger, well designed randomized studies to standardize these predictive factors for children. Also, the necessity for general anesthesia for endoscopic sessions in children is another worrying point. The deleterious effect of general anesthesia on the neurodevelopment of children is well documented. [33] And the recurrence of esophageal varices after eradication is common if the underlying cause of portal hypertension is not treated. There is increased incidence of gastric varices and portal hypertensive gastropathy after eradication of esophageal varices. The same is true regarding the non-selective beta-blocker. There is no properly designed randomized study to assess the therapeutic doses and the safety of the drug in children [34]. Taking into account the mortality rate due to the first variceal bleeding is exceedingly low (1%). All these points together came against standardizing the primary prophylaxis in children. But in special circumstances, the primary prophylaxis in children is justifiable like the child living away from the medical facilities which may necessitate primary prophylaxis.

9. Secondary prophylaxis

The secondary prophylaxis is the prevention of recurrence of variceal bleeding after the first variceal bleeding. Secondary prophylaxis is recommended in children due to the high recurrence rate after the first bleeding and enough data supporting the efficiency and safety of endoscopic banding and superior to endoscopic sclerotherapy therapy. As in the primary prophylaxis, no enough data support the safety and efficiency of non-selective beat-blockers. [28, 35]

10. Radiological intervention

TIPS refers to an establishment of intrahepatic portosystemic by inserting a stent (a communication) between the portal and hepatic veins. [36] It can be used in acute variceal bleeding uncontrolled by other means. Also, it is considered a good option for bridging to liver transplant for patients who have cirrhosis to improve the severe symptoms (e.g. Massive ascites). In this scenario, TIPS is considered an ideal option by avoiding abdominal operation with subsequent adhesions and fibrosis, which makes the liver transplant operation much easier. [26]

This technique is considered as a non-selective shunt where most of the portal blood diverted to the systemic circulation which participates in encephalopathy. Also, TIPS has potential complications, which are shunt stenosis/thrombosis, bleeding, and dislodge of the stent to the right atrium. [26, 34]

11. Surgical shunts

The type of surgery depends on the level of obstruction (pre-hepatic, hepatic. Post-hepatic).

Pre-hepatic portal vein thrombosis with suitable anatomy means a patent left portal vein in the umbilical fissure and the patent superior mesenteric vein. They connect via graft whether synthetic or autologous, but as a rule in pediatric surgery, the use of autologous graft is always preferred whenever it is possible due to the fact the graft grows with the child. The most used autologous graft is one of the internal jugular veins after making sure the contralateral one patent pre-operatively by doppler ultrasound. After the anastomosis has been established, the porto-systemic circulation is re-established. Another important point that the liver parenchyma in the extrahepatic portal thrombosis is preserved for a long time. Based on this fact the functionality of the liver is expected to recover after re-establishing the porto-systemic circulation. Fortunately, the data of the surgical outcome confirms this concept. The secondary coagulation abnormalities, hepatopulmonary syndrome, liver adenomas, encephalopathy, and neurocognitive all will be reverted after successful Rex shunt. [37] And for the congenital portosystemic shunt the surgical ligation of the shunt when it is technically feasible. [27]

When the cause of portal hypertension is liver cirrhosis in the modern era the suitable option is a liver transplant. [38]

There are other surgical options for portal hypertension which are considered palliative rather than therapeutic: (1) Selective shunt: the technique is known as distal splenorenal shunt (Warren shunt). The principle of this technique is diverting part of the portal circulation to the systemic circulation by dividing the splenic vein and anastomosing the distal end to the left renal vein. It helps to reduce gastro-esophageal variceal pressure subsequently reducing the bleeding potentials. Also, hypersplenism and encephalopathy are improved. But the issue with this shunt is that with time the selective shunt becomes non-selective due to the formation of collaterals. [26]

(2) Non-selective shunt: its principle is based on diverting the whole portal circulation to systemic circulation by mobilization of the superior mesenteric vein and creation of side to side anastomosis with inferior vena cava or by used graft to connect the 2 veins whether synthetic or autologous grafts. This technique is not preferred in children because of the high-risk encephalopathy and deleterious effect on the cognitive ability of the children. [38]

Author details

Reda A. Zbaida
Pediatric Surgery Department, Stellenbosch University, Cape Town, South Africa

*Address all correspondence to: redazbida@yahoo.co.uk

References

[1] Merkel C, Montagnese S. Hepatic venous pressure gradient measurement in clinical hepatology. Dig Liver Dis. 2011;43(10):762-7.

[2] Shneider BL, Bosch J, De Franchis R, Emre SH, Groszmann RJ, Ling SC, et al. Portal hypertension in children: Expert pediatric opinion on the report of the Baveno v consensus workshop on methodology of diagnosis and therapy in portal hypertension. Pediatr Transplant. 2012;16(5):426-37.

[3] Embryology G, Embryology S. part one General Embryology. Langman'S Med Embryol. :300-4.

[4] Collardeau-Frachon S, Scoazec JY. Vascular development and differentiation during human liver organogenesis. Anat Rec. 2008;291(6):614-27.

[5] Juza RM, Pauli EM. Clinical and surgical anatomy of the liver: A review for clinicians. Clin Anat. 2014;27(5):764-9.

[6] John E. Skandalakis et al., Surg Clin N Am 84 (2004) 413-435

[7] Mahadevan V. Anatomy of the liver. Surg (United Kingdom) [Internet]. 2020;38(8):427-31. Available from: http://dx.doi.org/10.1016/j.mpsur.2014.10.004

[8] LAWRENCE E. WINESKI P. Snell's clinical anatomy by Regions. Vol. 53, Wolters Kluwer. 2019. 2019 p.

[9] Abd El-Hamid N, Taylor RM, Marinello D, Mufti GJ, Patel R, Mieli-Vergani G, et al. Aetiology and management of extrahepatic portal vein obstruction in children: king's college hospital experience. J Pediatr Gastroenterol Nutr. 2008;47(5):630-4.

[10] Weiss B, Shteyer E, Vivante A, Berkowitz D, Reif S, Weizman Z, et al. Etiology and long-term outcome of extrahepatic portal vein obstruction in children. World J Gastroenterol. 2010;16(39):4968-72.

[11] Lautz TB, Tantemsapya N, Rowell E, Superina RA. Management and classification of type II congenital portosystemic shunts. J Pediatr Surg [Internet]. 2011;46(2):308-14. Available from: http://dx.doi.org/10.1016/j.jpedsurg.2010.11.009

[12] Chapin CA, Bass LM. Cirrhosis and Portal Hypertension in the Pediatric Population. Clin Liver Dis [Internet]. 2018;22(4):735-52. Available from: https://doi.org/10.1016/j.cld.2018.06.007

[13] Cesaro S, Pillon M, Talenti E, Toffolutti T, Calore E, Tridello G, et al. A prospective survey on incidence, risk factors and therapy of hepatic veno-occlusive disease in children after hematopoietic stem cell transplantation. Haematologica. 2005;90(10):1396-404.

[14] Nobre S, Khanna R, Bab N, Kyrana E, Height S, Karani J, et al. Primary Budd-Chiari Syndrome in Children: King's College Hospital Experience. J Pediatr Gastroenterol Nutr. 2017;65(1):93-6.

[15] Duché M, Ducot B, Ackermann O, Guérin F, Jacquemin E, Bernard O. Portal hypertension in children: High-risk varices, primary prophylaxis and consequences of bleeding. J Hepatol. 2017;66(2):320-7.

[16] El-Rifai N, Mention K, Guimber D, Michaud L, Boman F, Turck D, et al. Gastropathy and gastritis in children with portal hypertension. J Pediatr Gastroenterol Nutr. 2007;45(1):137-40.

[17] Gugig R, Rosenthal P. Management of portal hypertension in children. World J Gastroenterol. 2012;18(11):1176-84.

[18] Alvarez F, Bernard O, Brunelle F, Hadchouel M, Leblanc A, Odièvre M, et al. Congenital hepatic fibrosis in children. J Pediatr. 1981;99(3):370-5.

[19] D'Antiga L, Dacchille P, Boniver C, Poledri S, Schiff S, Zancan L, et al. Clues for minimal hepatic encephalopathy in children with noncirrhotic portal hypertension. J Pediatr Gastroenterol Nutr. 2014;59(6):689-94.

[20] Cosarderelioglu C, Cosar AM, Gurakar M, Pustavoitau A, Russell SD, Dagher NN, et al. Portopulmonary hypertension and liver transplant: Recent review of the literature. Exp Clin Transplant. 2016;14(2):113-20.

[21] Karrer FM, Wallace BJ, Estrada AE. Late complications of biliary atresia: hepatopulmonary syndrome and portopulmonary hypertension. Pediatr Surg Int [Internet]. 2017;33(12):1335-40. Available from: http://dx.doi.org/10.1007/s00383-017-4176-2

[22] Bavdekar A, Thakur N. Ascites in Children. Indian J Pediatr [Internet]. 2016;83(11):1334-40. Available from: http://dx.doi.org/10.1007/s12098-016-2168-1

[23] Rodwell VW. Harper's Illustrated Biochemistery. McGraw-Hill Eduction: Thrity-Fir; 2018

[24] Robson SC, Kahn D, Kruskal J, Bird AR, Kirsch RE. Disordered hemostasis in extrahepatic portal hypertension. Hepatology. 1993;18(4):853-7.

[25] D'Antiga L. Medical management of esophageal varices and portal hypertension in children. Semin Pediatr Surg [Internet]. 2012;21(3):211-8. Available from: http://dx.doi.org/10.1053/j.sempedsurg.2012.05.004

[26] de Ville de Goyet J, D'Ambrosio G, Grimaldi C. Surgical management of portal hypertension in children. Semin Pediatr Surg [Internet]. 2012;21(3):219-32. Available from: http://dx.doi.org/10.1053/j.sempedsurg.2012.05.005

[27] Guérin F, Blanc T, Gauthier F, Abella SF, Branchereau S. Congenital portosystemic vascular malformations. Semin Pediatr Surg [Internet]. 2012;21(3):233-44. Available from: http://dx.doi.org/10.1053/j.sempedsurg.2012.05.006

[28] Shneider BL, de Ville de Goyet J, Leung DH, Srivastava A, Ling SC, Duché M, et al. Primary prophylaxis of variceal bleeding in children and the role of MesoRex Bypass: Summary of the Baveno VI Pediatric Satellite Symposium. Hepatology. 2016;63(4):1368-80.

[29] Eroglu Y, Emerick KM, Whitingon PF, Alonso EM. Octreotide therapy for control of acute gastrointestinal bleeding in children. J Pediatr Gastroenterol Nutr. 2004;38(1):41-7.

[30] Altraif I, Handoo FA, Aljumah A, Alalwan A, Dafalla M, Saeed AM, et al. Effect of erythromycin before endoscopy in patients presenting with variceal bleeding: A prospective, randomized, double-blind, placebo-controlled trial. Gastrointest Endosc [Internet]. 2011;73(2):245-50. Available from: http://dx.doi.org/10.1016/j.gie.2010.09.043

[31] Bari K, Garcia-Tsao G. Treatment of portal hypertension. World J Gastroenterol. 2012;18(11):1166-75.

[32] North American Symptomatic Carotid Endarterectomy Trial Collaborators. The New England Journal of Medicine Downloaded from nejm.org at INSERM DISC DOC on October 6, 2015. For personal use only. No other uses without permission. Copyright © 1991 Massachusetts Medical Society. All rights reserved. N Engl J Med. 1991;325:445-53.

[33] Wang X, Xu Z, Miao CH. Current clinical evidence on the effect of general anesthesia on neurodevelopment in children: An updated systematic review with meta-regression. PLoS One. 2014;9(1).

[34] Bozic MA, Puri K, Molleston JP. Screening and Prophylaxis for Varices in Children with Liver Disease. Curr Gastroenterol Rep. 2015;17(7).

[35] Dos Santos JMR, Ferreira AR, Fagundes EDT, Ferreira APS, Ferreira LS, Magalhães MCR, et al. Endoscopic and pharmacological secondary prophylaxis in children and adolescents with esophageal varices. J Pediatr Gastroenterol Nutr. 2013;56(1):93-8.

[36] Di Giorgio A, Agazzi R, Alberti D, Colledan M, D'Antiga L. Feasibility and efficacy of transjugular intrahepatic portosystemic shunt (TIPS) in children. J Pediatr Gastroenterol Nutr. 2012;54(5):594-600.

[37] Di Francesco F, Grimaldi C, De Ville De Goyet J. Meso-Rex bypass - A procedure to cure prehepatic portal hypertension: The insight and the inside. J Am Coll Surg [Internet]. 2014;218(2):e23-36. Available from: http://dx.doi.org/10.1016/j.jamcollsurg.2013.10.024

[38] Scholz S, Sharif K. Surgery for portal hypertension in children. Curr Gastroenterol Rep. 2011;13(3):279-85.

Chapter 3

Sinusoidal Obstruction Syndrome

Yanxia Fei, Yanhua Peng, Huiping Sun, Shuangfa Zou and Jinfeng Yang

Abstract

Sinusoidal obstructive syndrome (SOS) is a fibrous occlusive disease of hepatic sinusoids or hepatic venules. Small hepatic blood vessel damage, especially hepatic sinusoidal endothelial cell damage, is its main feature. Based on etiology, SOS is mainly classified into pyrrolidine alkaloids-related SOS, hematopoietic stem cell transplantation-related SOS, and SOS of unknown etiology. In recent years, the incidence of SOS has been increasing. However, due to the complexity of the etiology, the lack of specificity in clinical manifestations, the difficulty of early diagnosis, and the limited treatment options, it often leads to poor treatment effects and even death. This chapter aims to analyze and organize the pathogenesis, pathological characteristics, diagnosis, treatment, and prognosis of different types of SOS, to provide certain references for the prevention and treatment of the disease.

Keywords: sinusoidal obstructions syndrome, hepatic vascular endothelial injury, hepatic venous pressure gradient, nonportal cirrhosis, pyrrolidine alkaloids-related SOS, hematopoietic stem cell transplantation-related SOS

1. Introduction

Hepatic sinusoidal obstruction syndrome (SOS), formerly known as a hepatic veno-occlusive disease (HVOD), is an intrahepatic hepatic sinusoidal portal hypertension caused by obstruction of the hepatic sinusoidal outflow tract due to endothelial cell injury. The main features of SOS are luminal narrowing or occlusion due to endothelial cell injury of the hepatic blood sinusoids, small hepatic veins, and interlobular veins. This causes intrahepatic stasis, hepatic injury and intrahepatic sinusoidal portal hypertension as a characteristic hepatic vasculogenic disease. Its clinical manifestations are mainly pain in the liver area, jaundice, ascites and hepatomegaly. The first cases were documented in South Africa in 1920 when cirrhosis was thought to be caused by groundsel poisoning [1]. In 1953, Hill et al. reported that more than 100 Jamaican children developed "Serous Hepatosis" from the consumption of Senecio (also known as groundsel) [2]. In 1954, Bras and Jelliffe et al. used the term hepatic veno-occlusive disease (HVOD) in their report [3]. Since then, with the recognition of HVOD, in 2002, Deleve et al. suggested that it would be more appropriately named SOS [4, 5], which is now generally accepted and adopted by scholars. The etiology of SOS is diverse, with different etiologies in China and Western countries. Depending on the etiology, it is mainly divided into hematopoietic stem cell transplantation-induced SOS (HSCT-SOS) and pyrrolidine alkaloids-induced SOS (PA-SOS). In the West, SOS is usually associated with myeloablative pretreatment before HSCT, and the incidence of HSCT-SOS ranges from 5.3% to 13.7% [6], even up to 60% in pediatric high-risk populations [7–9], and is an important complication and major obstacle of HSCT. In China, on the other hand, SOS is usually associated with oral intake of plants containing PA, with 50.0% to 88.6% of SOS caused by the consumption of sedum Tusanqi [10]. In recent years, the incidence of SOS has been increasing, but the complex etiology, lack of specificity of clinical manifestations, difficulties in early diagnosis and limited therapeutic means often lead to poor treatment outcomes and even death. The mortality rate of patients with multiple organ failure is greater than 80% [11]. However, the pathogenesis of the disease is not known. The existing guidelines are limited to "the SOS associated with hematopoietic stem cell transplantation in Western countries" and the "Nanjing criteria" developed by the Hepatobiliary Diseases Committee of the Chinese Society of Gastroenterology to diagnose and treatment of PA–HSOS [12, 13]. To this end, this section focuses on the research progress in the pathogenesis, clinical manifestations, diagnosis, treatment, prognosis, and preventive measures of SOS.

2. Etiology

2.1 Hematopoietic stem cell transplantation

HSCT is considered a major etiology of SOS in the West and is associated with high-dose chemotherapeutic drug pretreatment. Also, age, type of transplantation, secondary transplantation, cytokines produced by damaged tissues, endogenous microorganisms translocated by damaged mucosal barriers, immune factors, previous history of liver disease, systemic irradiation, local procoagulant status, and platelet adhesion are also risk factors for the development of HSCT-SOS [14–16].

2.2 Consumption of plants containing pyrrolidine alkaloids (PA)

In developing countries, such as China, Southeast Asian countries, and African countries, SOS is mainly caused by the consumption of plants containing PA. Plants containing PA are widely distributed around the world, and more than 300 of the more than 6000 species of plants are known to contain PA. For example, senecio, Tusanqi, lily, retrorsine, comfrey, etc. [17]. Since Chinese herbal medicine is widely used in China, SOS is mainly caused by poisoning with Tusanqi [18, 19]. In 1980, Hou et al. [20] reported for the first time two clinical cases of SOS caused by the administration of Tusanqi in China, which attracted widespread attention of clinicians, and since then, cases of SOS caused by Tusanqi have been reported throughout the country. PA and its hydrolysis products are not toxic, but when they reach the liver, they are deoxygenated by cytochrome P450 enzyme (CYP) 3A to form pyrrole-like derivatives. This metabolite binds to DNA/RNA in hepatocytes, thus affecting protein synthesis and inhibiting cell division, which in turn causes severe damage to the liver [21].

2.3 After radiation and chemotherapy

In addition to the above two common types, it has also been reported that SOS is associated with chemotherapy and radiotherapy for solid tumors, such as chemotherapy with cyclophosphamide. Common SOS-related drugs are cyclophosphamide, busulfan, dacarbazine, 6-mercaptopurine, 6-thioguanine, dacarbazine, actinomycin D, gemtuzumab, melphalan, oxaliplatin, cytarabine, and uratan [21].

2.4 After immune drug treatment

Recent reports say that SOS is associated with the use of immunosuppressive drugs [22]. As in the case of treatment with immunosuppressive agents after orthotopic liver transplantation, immune dysregulation is a direct cause of induction of SOS. Thus the indications for immunosuppressive agents, including azathioprine, also seem to be risk factors for SOS. This makes it difficult for researchers to establish the relationship between SOS and immunosuppression. Researchers believe that immune-related injury-induced damage is related to the pathogenesis of these rare lesions.

3. Pathological mechanism

The hepatic sinusoids are small vessels that constitute the hepatic microcirculation and are composed of hepatic sinusoidal endothelial cells (SEC) while being restricted by hepatic stellate cells. Therefore, the permeability of hepatic sinusoids is large, which facilitates the exchange of substances between hepatocytes and blood flow. When SOS occurs sinusoidal endothelial cells are damaged and shed, then migrate to the central veins of the hepatic lobules, leading to the formation of centripetal non-thrombotic obstruction of the hepatic sinusoids and central veins. Subsequently, coupled with the accumulation of erythrocytes and non-cellular debris, the formation of thrombus is another important factor that disrupts hepatic microcirculation and increases hepatic vascular resistance. A cascade of actions and interactions, as well as activation of exo-clotting factors, oxidative stress, and altered vascular permeability, all contributes to varying degrees to the obstruction of normal blood flow and increased venous resistance. This ultimately leads to portal hypertension, hepatic dysfunction and ascites retention [23] (**Figure 1**). Damage to SEC is manifested by intracellular glutathione depletion, decreased nitric oxide, and increased expression of matrix metalloproteinase (MMP) and vascular endothelial growth factor (VEGF). In addition to this, cytokines secreted by

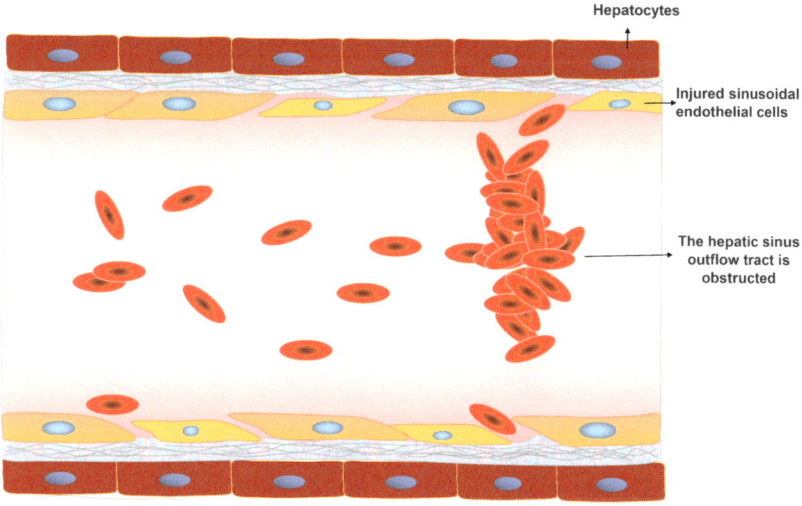

Figure 1.
Snusoidal obstruction syndrome (SOS) pathogenesis. Damage to the endothelial cells of the hepatic sinusoids due to HSCT or PA, etc. → blockage of the hepatic sinusoidal outflow tract → damage to the endothelial cells of the small and central hepatic veins → portal hypertension.

the damaged SEC lead to a weakened mucosal barrier between cells. This promotes the escape of erythrocytes, leukocytes, and platelets between hepatocytes and hepatic sinusoidal SEC, contributing to the initiation of inflammatory processes and thrombus formation [24, 25].

In HSCT-SOS, patients receiving high doses of toxic drugs (e.g., cyclophosphamide and leucovorin) during treatment are the cause of initial endothelial cell injury, which can lead to SOS, graft-versus-host disease (GVHD), capillary leak syndrome, implantation syndrome, and diffuse alveolar hemorrhage [26, 27]. In PA-SOS, the typical pathological changes are swelling, injury, and detachment of SEC in zone III of the hepatic acinus. The predominance of lesions in zone III of the hepatic acinus in PA-SOS is due to the abundance of CYP3A and the relative lack of glutathione (GSH) in this region. By constructing an animal model, Deleve et al. found that early damage to the endothelium of the hepatic sinusoids and central veins occurred before the development of veno-occlusive lesions, and that coagulative necrosis of hepatocytes occurred later than endothelial damage [3]. Besides, Harb et al. found that bone marrow progenitor cells were able to replace endothelial cells and thus repair the injury, while monocrotaline was able to inhibit endothelial progenitor cells in the bone marrow and circulation [28]. Therefore, PA damage to bone marrow progenitor cells and thus inhibition of endothelial cell repair may be another important pathogenetic mechanism. When SOS occurs, the hepatic sinusoidal stasis and dilatation; hepatic cord compression and atrophy; hepatocyte degeneration and necrosis; and central small vein occlusion and fibrosis are seen under light microscopy [29].

4. Clinical presentation

The main symptoms of SOS are non-specific: with or without ascites, pain, hepatomegaly, and jaundice. Clinical manifestations range from very few symptoms to multi-organ failure leading to patient death. The clinical manifestations of HSCT-SOS and PA-SOS differ in several aspects.

HSCT-SOS usually presents with abdominal distention, hepatomegaly, pain in the liver area, ascites, jaundice, loss of appetite, and weakness [30]. HSCT-SOS has a rapid onset, usually occurring within 21 d after bone marrow transplantation. And the proportion of seriously ill patients and mortality is high, most of them die from multi-organ dysfunction syndrome and sepsis [11]. A European multicenter study [6] graded SOS according to the severity of the disease: mild (about 8%) is self-limiting and recovers without special treatment; moderate (about 64%) recovers with aggressive treatment, and severe (about 28%) often leads to death because of progression, or no improvement after 100 d of treatment. In 2016, the European Society for Blood and Marrow Transplantation updated the HSCT-SOS scale, as shown in **Table 1** [26]. Due to the marked differences in incidence, genetic susceptibility, clinical presentation, prevention, treatment, and outcome between age groups, the European Society for Blood and Marrow Transplantation proposed new criteria specifically for SOS/VOD in children in 2018, as shown in **Table 2** [31].

PA-SOS mainly presents with abdominal distention and ascites [32], only about half of the patients present with hepatomegaly or jaundice, and a few patients have hepatoceles [33]. Most patients with PA-SOS have insignificant elevations in serum alanine aminotransferase, serum aspartate aminotransferase, alkaline phosphatase, γ-glutamyl transferase, and total bilirubin levels. PA-SOS occurs after a variable incubation period, which is usually about 30 d after drug administration and maybe up to several years. It can develop in both children and adults. In addition, PA-SOS

	Mild	*Moderate*	*Sever*	*Very sever -MOD/MOF*
Time since first clinical symptoms of SOS/VOD	>7 Days	5–7 Days	≤4 Days	Any time
Bilirubin (mg/dL) Bilirubin (μmol/L)	≥2 and < 3 ≥34 and < 51	≥3 and < 5 ≥51 and < 85	≥5 and < 8 ≥85 and < 136	≥8 ≥136
Bilirubin kinetics			Doubling within 48 h	
Transaminases	≤2 × normal	>2 and ≤5 × normal	45 and ≤8 × normal	48 × Normal
Weight increase	< 5%	≥5% and < 10%	≥5% and < 10%	≥10%
Renal function (baseline at transplant)	<1.2	≥ 1.2 and < 1.5	≥1.5 and < 2	≥2 or others signs of MOD/MOF

EBMT, European society for Blood and Marrow Transplantation; MDO, multi-organ dysfunction; MOF, multi-organ failure; SOS, sinusoidal obstruction syndrome; VOD, veno-occlusive disease.

Table 1.
New EBMT criteria for severity grading of a suspected SOS/VOD in adults.

	Mild	*Moderate*	*Sever*	*Very sever -MOD/MOF*
LFT (ALT, AST, GLDH)	≤2 × normal	>2 and ≤5 × normal	>5	
Persistent RT	< 3 days	3–7 days	> 7 days	
Bilirubin (mg/dL) Bilirubin (μmol/L)	< 2 < 34		≥ 2 ≥ 34	
Ascites	Minimal	Moderate	Necessity for paracentesis (external drainage)	
Bilirubin kinetics				Doubling within 48 h
Coagulation	Normal	Normal	Impaired coagulation	Impaired coagulation with need for replacement of coagulation factors
Renal function GFR (mL/min)	89–60	59–30	29–15	<15(renal failure)
Pulmonary function (oxygen requirement)	< 2 L/min	< 2 L/min	Invasive pulmonary ventilation (including CPAP)	
CNS	Normal	Normal	Normal	New onset cognitive impairment

EBMT, European society for Blood and Marrow Transplantation; ALT, alanine transaminase; AST, aspartate transaminase; CNS, central nervous system; CPAP, continuous positive airway pressure; CTCAE, Common Terminology Criteria for Adverse Events; GFR, glomerular filtration rate; GLDH, glutamate dehydrogenase; LFT, liver function test; MOD/MOF, multi-organ dysfunction/multi-organ failure; RT, refractory thrombocytopenia; SOS/VOD, sinusoidal obstruction syndrome/veno-occlusive disease.

Table 2.
EBMT criteria for grading the severity of suspected hepatic SOS/VOD in children.

has a lower rate of severe disease than HSCT-SOS [34, 35], and mortality is generally around 40%, with most deaths due to progressive liver failure and infection [36, 37]. Since PA-SOS is associated with extensive fibrosis in the central region of the lobules and histological examination shows venous-centered cirrhosis, it is difficult to distinguish from other causes of chronic lesions of cirrhosis.

5. Diagnosis

5.1 Symptoms and signs

Pain in the liver area, hepatomegaly, jaundice, ascites, and significant weight gain in a short period are more common.

5.2 Pathology

The biopsy is the gold standard for confirming the diagnosis of SOS. Liver histology is characterized by bruising of the liver tissue, dilatation of the hepatic sinusoids, swelling and damage to the endothelial cells of the hepatic sinusoids, and shedding. In particular, the thickening, fibrosis, luminal narrowing, and even occlusion of small hepatic veins are typical of the disease. However, hepatic stasis and swelling are associated with a high risk of puncture and can be falsely negative due to heterogeneous intrahepatic lesions.

5.3 Laboratory tests

Serum total bilirubin (TBil) or other liver functions (alanine aminotransferase, aspartate aminotransferase, total bile acids, and albumin).

5.4 Radiographic examinations

Ultrasonography shows a thin inner diameter of the hepatic vein (< 5 mm) with a smooth lining and luminal patency and a slowed flow velocity in the hepatic vein (< 20 cm/s). This is different from hepatic vein stenosis (Bard-Chiari syndrome). Also, the hepatic sinusoids and small venous lesions are not uniformly distributed within the liver in patients with SOS. As a result, areas of tissue bruising and necrosis may be distributed in a map-like fashion and appear on ultrasound images as heterogeneous intrahepatic echogenicity. Enhanced CT or MRI of the abdomen has diagnostic value, shows that the contrast in the portal and delayed phases is obstructed at the end of the portal branches and fails to enter the hepatic lobe segmental veins, resulting in unrepresented hepatic veins.

5.5 Hepatic venous pressure gradient measurement

The difference between free hepatic venous pressure and wedge pressure is the "hepatic venous pressure gradient (HVPG), measured by puncture of the internal jugular or femoral vein. When HVPG >5 mmHg, it indicates the presence of portal hypertension in cirrhosis. When HVPG >10 mmHg, the diagnostic specificity of SOS is 91%, and the chance of esophagogastric variceal bleeding and seroperitoneum will be greatly increased. The internationally recognized diagnostic criteria for HSCT-SOS are Seattle criteria, Baltimore criteria [38], and pediatric criteria [31], and PA-SOS diagnosis is mainly based on Nanjing criteria [13]. Several accepted diagnostic criteria are listed in **Table 3**.

DOI: http://dx.doi.org/10.5772/intechopen.96370

HSCT—SOS			*PA—SOS*
Seattle criteria	**Baltimore criteria**	**criteria for children**	**Nanjing criteria**
2 of the following 3 items within 20 d after bone marrow HSCT: • Serum TBil ≥34.2 umol/L; • Hepatomegaly or pain in the liver area; • Ascites or weight gain exceeding 2% of the original.	Serum TBil ≥34.2 pmo/L and within 21 d after bone marrow HSCT, 2 of the following 3 items were present simultaneously: • Hepatomegaly with hepatic pain; • Weight gain more than 5% of the original; • Ascites.	The presence of two or more of the followinga: • Onexplained consumptive and transfusion-refractory thrombocytopeniab; • Otherwise unexplained weight gain on three consecutive days despite the use of diuretics or a weight gain 45% above baseline value; • Hepatomegaly (best if confirmed by imaging) above baseline value; • Ascites (best if confirmed by imaging) above baseline value; • Rising bilirubin from a baseline value on 3 consecutive days or bilirubin ⩾2 mg/dL within 72 h.	Have a clear history of PA-containing plant consumption, while excluding other known causes of liver injury, and present with 3 of the following or confirmed by pathology: • Abdominal distention and/or pain in the liver region, hepatomegaly and ascites; • Elevated serum TBil or other liver function abnormalities; • Typical enhanced CT or MRI presentation. The diagnosis was confirmed by pathology with the following typical pathological findings: swelling, damage, and loss of endothelial cells in the hepatic sinusoids of zone III of the hepatic acinus, and significant dilatation and congestion of the hepatic sinusoids.

SOS, sinusoidal obstruction syndrome; HSCT-SOS, hematopoietic stem cell transplantation-induced SOS; PA-SOS, pyrrolidine alkaloids-induced SOS; CT, computed tomography; MIR, magnetic resonance imaging.

Table 3.
Diagnostic criteria for hepatic SOS.

6. Treatment

The principles of treatment for SOS include discontinuing the use of plants containing PA in suspected patients and starting symptomatic and supportive treatment as soon as possible.

6.1 symptomatic and supportive treatment

Symptomatic and supportive treatment is particularly important for patients in the acute or subacute phase, including hepatoprotection, diuresis, nutritional support, protein and vitamin supplementation, and improvement of microcirculation. Oral furosemide and spironolactone are preferred as diuretics. If ascites are severe and not responding to pharmacological therapy, peritoneal drainage may be considered. For patients with fluid retention and severe renal failure, hemodialysis or hemofiltration should be performed. Patients with multiple organ failures should be admitted to the intensive care unit. In most patients, symptomatic and supportive treatment can reduce water-sodium retention, repair damaged hepatocytes, and promote recovery of liver function, but it cannot significantly reverse pathophysiological changes and needs to be combined with other treatments together [39].

6.2 Anticoagulant therapy

For patients in the acute or subacute phase, anticoagulation should be started as early as possible unless there are contraindications (including severe bleeding or bleeding tendency). The preferred choice is low-molecular-weight heparin at the recommended dose of 100 IU/kg, administered subcutaneously every 12 hours. In China, the cure rate of patients with PA-SOS treated with low-molecular heparin in the past was up to 70.7–88.9% [40–43]. Monitoring is not required in most patients because of the low side effects of low molecular heparin, but it should be used with caution in patients with renal failure. Oral warfarin, the oral anticoagulant of choice for long-term treatment, can also be administered. Its efficacy is evaluated by monitoring the international standardized ratio of prothrombin time (recommended 2.0 to 3.0). However, warfarin therapy has a narrow dose range, a wide variation in individual response, and a vulnerability to various food and drug interactions for efficacy. An imageological should be performed after 2 weeks of anticoagulation therapy, and clinical manifestations and liver function should be evaluated. If treatment is effective, anticoagulation therapy can be continued for up to 3 months. Conversely, if it is ineffective, treatment should be discontinued and alternative therapies may be considered.

6.3 Glucocorticoid

High-dose hormone therapy may be efficacious for HSCT-SOS, but the risk of infection is a concern and the level of evidence is low. The efficacy of glucocorticoid therapy for PA-SOS is also controversial [12, 44–46].

6.4 Defibrotide

Defibrotide (DF) is an effective drug for the prevention and treatment of HSCT-SOS and can be used to treat severe HSCT-HSOS [12]. DF has anti-ischemic, anti-inflammatory, anti-thrombotic, and thrombolytic activities as well as protecting the small vessel endothelium and inhibiting fibrin deposition. The mechanism may be the protection of endothelial cells and the maintenance of thrombus-fibrinolytic balance. However, the effectiveness of DF has not been tested in PA-SOS because its use for the treatment of SOS has not yet been approved in China.

6.5 Interventional therapy

Transjugular intrahepatic portosystemic shunt (TIPS) can be performed when medical treatment is ineffective. TIPS is effective in reducing portal pressure, improving clinical symptoms (ascites, hepatic distension, etc.), and preventing esophagogastric variceal hemorrhage [47]. TIPS is effective in patients with PA-SOS who have failed symptomatic treatment and require management of ascites and portal hypertension [48]. However, TIPS for acute HSCT-SOS has had variable results in one case report, with 5 of 10 patients dying after 10 days of TIPS placement, but the other 5 patients recovering significantly [49]. We need a longer follow-up to determine whether TIPS improves patient prognosis.

6.6 Liver transplantation

Liver transplantation is an effective treatment for various end-stage liver diseases, and it can be considered in patients with liver failure who have failed after the above treatments. Liver transplantation has been reported to improve the prognosis of patients with HSCT-SOS, but there are fewer reports on PA-SOS [38].

6.7 Other

Antithrombin III [50], recombinant human soluble thrombomodulin [51], N-acetyl-L-cysteine [52], and recombinant human tissue-plasminogen activator (t-PA) [53] have also been studied and reported for the treatment of HSCT-SOS. However, the efficacy of these drugs is unknown, and they lack evidence in the treatment of PA-SOS.

Prognosis: The overall morbidity and mortality rate is 20% to 50%. Mild paticnts heal better; most moderate patients can improve after symptomatic management and other treatments, and the morbidity and mortality rate is about 25%; severe patients are often complicated by multi-organ failure and have a morbidity and mortality rate of more than 90% despite active treatment [54].

7. Conclusion

In conclusion, there is no specific treatment for SOS and the prognosis of patients is poor, and only liver transplantation can prolong the survival time of patients with advanced disease. Therefore, the emphasis is on prevention, including pretreatment of transplantation and early treatment of underlying blood disorders to decrease the incidence and severity of HSCT-SOS, and increasing awareness of Chinese herbs such as Tusanqi to avoid accidental ingestion to reduce the incidence of PA-SOS. Besides, early diagnosis and assessment of patient risk through biomarkers is an effective tool for disease prevention and management [55].

Acknowledgements

This work was financially supported by Hunan Provincial Natural Science Foundation of China (Grant No. 2020JJ4421 and 2019JJ80020 and 2019JJ40180).

Conflict of interest

The authors declare no conflict of interest.

Author details

Yanxia Fei, Yanhua Peng, Huiping Sun, Shuangfa Zou and Jinfeng Yang*
Hunan Cancer Hospital, The Affiliated Cancer Hospital of Xiangya School of Medicine, Central South University, Changsha, Hunan, China

*Address all correspondence to: yangjinfeng@hnca.org.cn

References

[1] Lédinghen V de, Villate A, Robin M, et al. Sinusoidal obstruction syndrome[J]. Clinics and research in hepatology and gastroenterology, 2020, 44(4):480-485. DOI: 10.1016/j.clinre.2020.03.019.

[2] Hill K R, Rhodes K, Stafford J L, et al. Serous hepatosis: a pathogenesis of hepatic fibrosis in Jamaican children[J]. British medical journal, 1953, 1(4802):117-122. DOI: 10.1136/bmj.1.4802.117.

[3] Bras G, Jelliffe D B, Stuart K L. Veno-occlusive disease of liver with nonportal type of cirrhosis, occurring in Jamaica[J]. A.M.A. archives of pathology, 1954, 57(4):285-300.

[4] DeLeve L D, McCuskey R S, Wang X, et al. Characterization of a reproducible rat model of hepatic veno-occlusive disease[J]. Hepatology (Baltimore, Md.), 1999, 29(6):1779-1791. DOI: 10.1002/hep.510290615.

[5] DeLeve L D, Shulman H M, McDonald G B. Toxic injury to hepatic sinusoids: sinusoidal obstruction syndrome (veno-occlusive disease) [J]. Seminars in liver disease, 2002, 22(1):27-42. DOI: 10.1055/s-2002-23204.

[6] Carreras E, Bertz H, Arcese W, et al. Incidence and outcome of hepatic veno-occlusive disease after blood or marrow transplantation: a prospective cohort study of the European Group for Blood and Marrow Transplantation. European Group for Blood and Marrow Transplantation Chronic Leukemia Working Party[J]. Blood, 1998, 92(10):3599-3604.

[7] Corbacioglu S, Cesaro S, Faraci M, et al. Defibrotide for prophylaxis of hepatic veno-occlusive disease in paediatric haemopoietic stem-cell transplantation: an open-label, phase 3, randomised controlled trial[J]. The Lancet, 2012, 379(9823):1301-1309. DOI: 10.1016/S0140-6736(11)61938-7.

[8] Barker C C, Butzner J D, Anderson R A, et al. Incidence, survival and risk factors for the development of veno-occlusive disease in pediatric hematopoietic stem cell transplant recipients[J]. Bone marrow transplantation, 2003, 32(1):79-87. DOI: 10.1038/sj.bmt.1704069.

[9] Cesaro S, Pillon M, Talenti E, et al. A prospective survey on incidence, risk factors and therapy of hepatic veno-occlusive disease in children after hematopoietic stem cell transplantation[J]. Haematologica, 2005, 90(10):1396-1404.

[10] Zhuge Y, Liu Y, Xie W, et al. Expert consensus on the clinical management of pyrrolizidine alkaloid-induced hepatic sinusoidal obstruction syndrome[J]. Journal of gastroenterology and hepatology, 2019, 34(4):634-642. DOI: 10.1111/jgh.14612.

[11] Coppell J A, Richardson P G, Soiffer R, et al. Hepatic veno-occlusive disease following stem cell transplantation: incidence, clinical course, and outcome[J]. Biology of blood and marrow transplantation: journal of the American Society for Blood and Marrow Transplantation, 2010, 16(2):157-168. DOI: 10.1016/j.bbmt.2009.08.024.

[12] Dignan F L, Wynn R F, Hadzic N, et al. BCSH/BSBMT guideline: diagnosis and management of veno-occlusive disease (sinusoidal obstruction syndrome) following haematopoietic stem cell transplantation[J]. British journal of haematology, 2013, 163(4):444-457. DOI: 10.1111/bjh.12558.

[13] Cooperative Group for Hepatic and Gall Diseases, Chinese Society of Gastroenterology, Chinese Medical

Association. Expert consensus on diagnosis and treatment of quinazoline alkaloids-related sinusoidal obstruction syndrome (2017 Nanjing) [J]. J Clin Hepatol, 2017, 33(9): 1627-1637. (in Chinese)

[14] Bonifazi F, Barbato F, Ravaioli F, et al. Diagnosis and Treatment of VOD/SOS After Allogeneic Hematopoietic Stem Cell Transplantation[J]. Frontiers in immunology, 2020, 11:489. DOI: 10.3389/fimmu.2020.00489.

[15] Devarbhavi H, Singh R, Patil M, et al. Outcome and determinants of mortality in 269 patients with combination anti-tuberculosis drug-induced liver injury[J]. Journal of gastroenterology and hepatology, 2013, 28(1):161-167. DOI: 10.1111/j.1440-1746.2012.07279.x.

[16] Kim J, Jung Y. Radiation-induced liver disease: current understanding and future perspectives[J]. Experimental & molecular medicine, 2017, 49(7): e359. DOI: 10.1038/emm.2017.85.

[17] Prakash A S, Pereira T N, Reilly P E, et al. Pyrrolizidine alkaloids in human diet[J]. Mutation research, 1999, 443(1-2):53-67. DOI: 10.1016/s1383-5742(99)00010-1.

[18] Wang X, Qi X, Guo X. Tusanqi-Related Sinusoidal Obstruction Syndrome in China: A Systematic Review of the Literatures[J]. Medicine, 2015, 94(23): e942. DOI: 10.1097/MD.0000000000000942.

[19] Hou J G. Veno-occlusive disease of the liver with report of 2 cases (author's transl) [J]. Zhonghua nei ke za zhi, 1980, 19(3):187-191.

[20] Yang M, Ruan J, Gao H, et al. First evidence of pyrrolizidine alkaloid N-oxide-induced hepatic sinusoidal obstruction syndrome in humans[J]. Archives of toxicology, 2017, 91(12):3913-3925. DOI: 10.1007/s00204-017-2013-y.

[21] Fulgenzi A, Ferrero M E. Defibrotide in the treatment of hepatic veno-occlusive disease[J]. Hepatic medicine: evidence and research, 2016, 8:105-113. DOI: 10.2147/HMER.S79243.

[22] Kiel P J, Vargo C A, Patel G P, et al. Possible correlation of sirolimus plasma concentration with sinusoidal obstructive syndrome of the liver in patients undergoing myeloablative allogeneic hematopoietic cell transplantation[J]. Pharmacotherapy,2012, 32(5):441-445. DOI: 10.1002/j.1875-9114.2012.01034.x.

[23] Valla D-C, Cazals-Hatem D. Sinusoidal obstruction syndrome[J]. Clinics and research in hepatology and gastroenterology, 2016, 40(4):378-385. DOI: 10.1016/j.clinre.2016.01.006.

[24] Eissner G, Multhoff G, Holler E. Influence of bacterial endotoxin on the allogenicity of human endothelial cells[J]. Bone marrow transplantation, 1998, 21(12):1286-1288. DOI: 10.1038/sj.bmt.1701264.

[25] Palomo M, Diaz-Ricart M, Carbo C, et al. Endothelial dysfunction after hematopoietic stem cell transplantation: role of the conditioning regimen and the type of transplantation[J]. Biology of blood and marrow transplantation: journal of the American Society for Blood and Marrow Transplantation, 2010, 16(7):985-993. DOI: 10.1016/j.bbmt.2010.02.008.

[26] Mohty M, Malard F, Abecassis M, et al. Revised diagnosis and severity criteria for sinusoidal obstruction syndrome/veno-occlusive disease in adult patients: a new classification from the European Society for Blood and Marrow Transplantation[J]. Bone marrow transplantation, 2016, 51(7):906-912. DOI: 10.1038/bmt.2016.130.

[27] DeLeve L D. Cellular target of cyclophosphamide toxicity in the murine liver: role of glutathione and site of metabolic activation[J]. Hepatology (Baltimore, Md.), 1996, 24(4):830-837. DOI: 10.1002/hep.510240414.

[28] Harb R, Xie G, Lutzko C, et al. Bone marrow progenitor cells repair rat hepatic sinusoidal endothelial cells after liver injury[J]. Gastroenterology, 2009, 137(2):704-712. DOI: 10.1053/j.gastro.2009.05.009.

[29] Zhang F, Zhou Y, Yang X, et al. Gynura Rhizoma containing pyrrolizidine alkaloids induces the hepatic sinusoidal obstruction syndrome in mice via upregulating fibrosis-related factors[J]. Acta pharmacologica Sinica, 2019, 40(6):781-789. DOI: 10.1038/s41401-018-0155-y.

[30] Dalle J-H, Giralt S A. Hepatic Veno-Occlusive Disease after Hematopoietic Stem Cell Transplantation: Risk Factors and Stratification, Prophylaxis, and Treatment[J]. Biology of blood and marrow transplantation: journal of the American Society for Blood and Marrow Transplantation, 2016, 22(3):400-409. DOI: 10.1016/j.bbmt.2015.09.024.

[31] Corbacioglu S, Carreras E, Ansari M, et al. Diagnosis and severity criteria for sinusoidal obstruction syndrome/veno-occlusive disease in pediatric patients: a new classification from the European society for blood and marrow transplantation[J]. Bone marrow transplantation, 2018, 53(2):138-145. DOI: 10.1038/bmt.2017.161.

[32] Wang Y, Qiao D, Li Y, et al. Risk factors for hepatic veno-occlusive disease caused by Gynura segetum: a retrospective study[J]. BMC gastroenterology, 2018, 18(1):156. DOI: 10.1186/s12876-018-0879-7.

[33] Ren XF, Zhuge YZ, Chen SY. Hepatobiliary Cooperative Group of Chinese Society of Gastroenterology. Gynura segetum-related hepatic sinusoidal obstruction syndrome: a national multicenter clinical study[J]. Zhonghua Xiaohua Zazhi, 2017, 37:523-529. (in Chinese)

[34] Chao N. How I treat sinusoidal obstruction syndrome[J]. Blood, 2014, 123(26):4023-4026. DOI: 10.1182/blood-2014-03-551630.

[35] Kalayoglu-Besisik S, Yenerel M N, Caliskan Y, et al. Time-related changes in the incidence, severity, and clinical outcome of hepatic veno-occlusive disease in hematopoietic stem cell transplantation patients during the past 10 years[J]. Transplantation proceedings, 2005, 37(5):2285-2289. DOI: 10.1016/j.transproceed.2005.03.025.

[36] Carreras E. How I manage sinusoidal obstruction syndrome after haematopoietic cell transplantation[J]. British journal of haematology, 2015, 168(4):481-491. DOI: 10.1111/bjh.13215.

[37] Zhou C-Z, Wang R-F, Lv W-F, et al. Transjugular intrahepatic portosystemic shunt for pyrrolizidine alkaloid-related hepatic sinusoidal obstruction syndrome[J]. World journal of gastroenterology, 2020, 26(24):3472-3483. DOI: 10.3748/wjg.v26.i24.3472.

[38] DeLeve L D, Valla D-C, Garcia-Tsao G. Vascular disorders of the liver[J]. Hepatology (Baltimore, Md.), 2009, 49(5):1729-1764. DOI: 10.1002/hep.22772.

[39] Wu X-j, Zhang K, Yu M-y, et al. Clinical analysis of four cases of hepatic veno-occlusive disease caused by Gynura segetum (Lour.) Merr[J]. Zhonghua Ganzangbing Zazhi, 2007, 15(2):151-153.

[40] Zhu WL, Chen SH, Chen WX et al. Clinical analysis of 50 cases of hepatic

veno-occlusive disease. Chin. J. Dig. 2012, 32: 620-624. (in Chinese)

[41] Chen S, Li CL, Gao YY. The diagnostic value of Doppler ultrasound in hepatic veno-occlusive disease. Chin. Med. Radio. 2010, 18: 154-156. (in Chinese)

[42] Xu XJ, Chen HT, Shan GD. Analysis of clinical practice in hepatic sinusoidal obstruction disease induced by Tusanqi. Chin. J. Crit. Care Med. (Electronic Edition) 2010, 03: 178-80. (in Chinese)

[43] Song Y, Fan YH. Clinical features of hepatic veno-occlusive disease induced by gynura root: analysis of 102 cases. J. Clin. Hepatol. 2011, 27: 496-499. (in Chinese)

[44] Zhu H, Chu Y, Huo J, et al. Effect of prednisone on transforming growth factor-β1, connective tissue growth factor, nuclear factor-κBp65 and tumor necrosis factor-α expression in a murine model of hepatic sinusoidal obstruction syndrome induced by Gynura segetum[J]. Hepatology research: the official journal of the Japan Society of Hepatology, 2011, 41(8):795-803. DOI: 10.1111/j.1872-034X.2011.00830.x.

[45] Zhang YT, Li S, Zhou DH et al. Clinical features of sinusoidal obstruction syndrome: an analysis of 35 cases and literature review. J.Clin. Hepatol. 2013, 29: 936-939. (in Chinese)

[46] Xu JM. A multi-center analysis of hepatic veno-occlusive disease in China. 11th CGC. HangZhou. 2011, 42-4 (in Chinese)

[47] La Rubia J de, Carral A, Montes H, et al. Successful treatment of hepatic veno-occlusive disease in a peripheral blood progenitor cell transplant patient with a transjugular intrahepatic portosystemic stent-shunt (TIPS)[J]. Haematologica, 1996, 81(6):536-539.

[48] Azoulay D, Castaing D, Lemoine A, et al. Transjugular intrahepatic portosystemic shunt (TIPS) for severe veno-occlusive disease of the liver following bone marrow transplantation[J]. Bone marrow transplantation, 2000, 25(9):987-992. DOI: 10.1038/sj.bmt.1702386.

[49] Chen S, Li CL, Gao YY. The diagnostic value of Doppler ultrasound in hepatic veno-occlusive disease. Chin. Med. Radio. 2010, 18: 154-156. (in Chinese)

[50] Xu XJ, Chen HT, Shan GD. Analysis of clinical practice in hepatic sinusoidal obstruction disease induced by Tusanqi. Chin. J. Crit. Care Med. (Electronic Edition) 2010, 03: 178-80. (in Chinese)

[51] Nakamura D, Yoshimitsu M, Kawada H, et al. Recombinant human soluble thrombomodulin for the treatment of hepatic sinusoidal obstructive syndrome post allogeneic hematopoietic SCT[J]. Bone marrow transplantation, 2012, 47(3):463-464. DOI: 10.1038/bmt.2011.103.

[52] Barkholt L, Remberger M, Hassan Z, et al. A prospective randomized study using N-acetyl-L-cysteine for early liver toxicity after allogeneic hematopoietic stem cell transplantation[J]. Bone marrow transplantation, 2008, 41(9):785-790. DOI: 10.1038/sj.bmt.1705969.

[53] Yoon J-H, Min W-S, Kim H-J, et al. Experiences of t-PA use in moderate-to-severe hepatic veno-occlusive disease after hematopoietic SCT: is it still reasonable to use t-PA?[J]. Bone marrow transplantation, 2013, 48(12):1562-1568. DOI: 10.1038/bmt.2013.101.

[54] Lu Junzhu, Zhan Jun. Research progress on sinusoidal obstruction

syndrome caused by drug-induced liver injury[J]. New Med, 2017,48(12):833-838. (in Chinese)

[55] Weischendorff S, Kielsen K, Sengeløv H, et al. Associations between levels of insulin-like growth factor 1 and sinusoidal obstruction syndrome after allogeneic haematopoietic stem cell transplantation[J]. Bone marrow transplantation, 2017, 52(6):863-869. DOI: 10.1038/bmt.2017.43.

Section 2

Pathogenesis of Portal Hypertension

Chapter 4

Endothelial Dysfunction and Systemic Inflammation in the Pathogenesis and Progression of Portal Hypertension

Elena Curakova Ristovska

Abstract

Hepatic and extrahepatic factors contribute to mortality related to liver cirrhosis and therefore much research is still to be done in order to understand the condition thoroughly and to possibly intervene in the process. It is considered that the currently applied prognostic scores are not ideal mortality predictors. On the other hand, recent scientific concepts have revealed the significant contributing role of endothelial dysfunction and of systemic inflammation in the pathogenesis of portal hypertension. Consequently, these concepts are inevitably leading towards proposing and validating new prognostic indicators in cirrhotic patients. Von-Willebrand factor as an indicator of endothelial dysfunction and C-reactive protein as a surrogate marker of systemic inflammation and several other parameters and biological markers have been emerging as a relevant and potentially useful prognostic indicators. Also, the coagulopathy associated to liver disease is in close relation with these entities and still an important research topic. Despite the promising data regarding their prognostic potential, additional research is needed in order to define and validate their value more precisely in clinical and prognostic settings.

Keywords: cirrhosis, portal hypertension, endothelial dysfunction, systemic inflammation, von-Willebrand factor, CRP, coagulopathy

1. Introduction

Liver cirrhosis represents the final stage of chronic liver disease which denotes reduced hepatic cell mass, formation of regenerative nodules and progressive fibrosis. The altered hepatic architecture leads to an impaired hepatic haemodynamics that manifests with portal hypertension (PH) and gradually leads to development of liver failure [1, 2]. PH is an accompanying condition of the natural course of chronic liver disease and a key factor underlying most of the complications that often determine the prognosis in these patients [3]. Although the development of PH has been mainly attributed to the elevated hydrostatic pressure due to increased vascular resistance, different perspectives have recently emerged regarding this topic. Endothelial dysfunction (ED), a state that indicates irregular function of the endothelial cell (EC), seems to have an important role in the increased vascular tone of the hepatic microcirculation [4, 5] and is an important factor involved in

IntechOpen

the development of PH [6]. It is also considered that elevated von Willebrand factor (vWF) contributes to the presence of a subtle hypercoagulable state that worsens the PH [7]. Chronic liver disease has also been related to many complex abnormalities in all segments of the haemostatic process. Moreover, the simultaneous impairment in the procoagulant and anticoagulant activity and the increased vWF concentration transform liver cirrhosis into a condition that is characterized by a globally rebalanced hemostasis [8].

2. Portal hypertension: definition, diagnostic criteria, clinical and prognostic significance

PH is an entity that indicates elevated hydrostatic pressure in the portal vein that initially occurs as a result of the structural abnormalities in the hepatic vasculature [6]. The increased vascular inflow which develops as a consequence of the splanchnic vasodilation and of the increased cardiac "output" also contribute in the progressivon of PH [9]. The main diagnostic criterion for PH is the presence of elevated hepatic venous pressure gradient (HVPG). HVPG denotes the pressure gradient between the so-called "wedged" pressure and the free pressure of the hepatic veins, which actually reflects the pressure gradient between the portal vein and the inferior vena cava. The HVPG value correlates with PH-related complications [10] and the HVPG measurement is used in therapeutic as well as in prognostic purposes [11]. Clinically significant portal hypertension is defined as the presence of HVPG ≥10 mmHg and it indicates an increased risk of complications and death associated with liver disease and an increased risk of hepatocellular carcinoma [12–15]. HVPG ≥12 mmHg carries an increased risk of variceal bleeding, and HVPG ≥20 mmHg is associated with poor clinical outcomes in cirrhotic patients [12–15]. The PH-related complications are often life-threatening conditions associated with high morbidity and mortality [3] and hence early diagnosis and appropriate treatment is essential for improving the prognosis in these patients [16]. Although HVPG measurement is the gold standard for determining the presence and extent of PH, this diagnostic procedure is not widely used in the everyday clinical practice. It is invasive, expensive and due to technical reasons in about 4% of patients it could be unsuccessful [17]. Consequently, these limitations also preclude the widespread use of the diagnostic and therapeutic algorithms that rely on pressure-based diagnostics. Therefore, the Baveno V Consensus for portal hypertension encourages research towards defining new, non-invasive indicators of PH with better sensitivity and specificity than the ones that are currently used [16, 18].

The natural course of chronic liver disease is characterized by two phases. The first compensated phase is followed by a rapidly progressing, decompensated phase characterized by the presence of complications of PH and/or hepatic dysfunction [1]. As the disease progresses, portal pressure increases and liver function decreases, leading to development of ascites, hypertensive gastrointestinal bleeding, encephalopathy, and jaundice [1]. The occurrence of any complication of PH defines the transition from a compensated to a decompensated phase [1]. The occurrence of ascites is the most common initial complication of PH in cirrhotic patients [19] and it is usually considered a hallmark of the decompensated phase [1]. By combining data from two large studies involving 1649 patients that analyzed the natural course of the disease [19, 20], four clinical stages of cirrhosis were defined, each with a different clinical presentation and a significantly different prognosis [1]. Stage 1 is characterized by the absence of esophageal varices and ascites (mortality rate about 1% per year); stage 2 is characterized by the presence of esophageal varices but without bleeding or ascites (mortality rate

3.4% per year); stage 3 is characterized by the presence of ascites with or without varices in a patient who has never bleed (mortality rate 20% per year) and stage 4 is characterized by gastrointestinal bleeding with or without ascites (mortality rate 57% per year). Stages 1 and 2 correspond to compensated and stages 3 and 4 to decompensated cirrhosis [1]. The transition from compensated to decompensated phase occurs at a rate of 5–7% per year [21, 22] and with the onset of the first episode of decompensation the life expectancy of patients is significantly shortened [1]. Median survival is significantly shorter in patients with decompensated than in patients with compensated cirrhosis (approximately 2 years versus over 12 years) [1]. Consequently, the prognostic indicators used in both stages are different and have different prognostic significance [23, 24].

3. The role of endothelial dysfunction in the pathogenesis of portal hypertension

EC has a potential for producing many different mediators that are crucial for proper regulation of the vascular homeostasis, the vasomotor tone and for many inflammatory, metabolic and hemostatic processes in the body [25]. EC regulates the vascular tone by its ability to release vasoactive substances, including vasodilators such as nitric oxide (NO) and prostacyclin and vasoconstrictors such as thromboxane A2 (TXA2) [9]. Endothelial activation is a broad term implying EC function changes occurring as a response to a number of different stimuli. As a response to vascular stress, infections or hypoxia, the EC undergoes certain changes that lead to an imbalance in the release of vasoactive mediators predisposing development of a pro-inflammatory and pro-coagulant state [26–32]. As a response to chronic, continuous exposure of the EC to various physical or chemical stimuli a disturbance in the function of the EC occurs, a state defined as ED. [25]. ED is a condition of imbalanced release of vasoconstrictors and vasodilators, stimulators and inhibitors of growth, proatherogenic and antiatherogenic, and pro-coagulant and anticoagulant mediators [4, 25]. It has been established that ED is an early key event in many vascular diseases [5] and its presence is generally associated with a poor prognosis [7]. Also, ED is an early event that has been involved in the pathogenesis of PH [6]. ED as part of the liver disease occurs in the liver microcirculation and in the EC in the systemic and splanchnic circulation. Hepatic inflammation in early cirrhosis is the primary trigger that causes damage to the hepatic reticuloendothelial system and leads to intrahepatic ED [33–41]. This ED is manifested by an increased release of vasoconstrictive substances leading to impaired flow-associated endothelial-dependent vascular relaxation, i.e., to inadequate postprandial vasodilation. Intrahepatic ED is considered to be the primary disorder that leads to increased intrahepatic vascular resistance and progressive PH [4, 5, 9, 42], and later, to a consequent arterial vasodilation in the splanchnic circulation [4, 43–45]. On the contrary, in advanced disease, endotoxemia is considered to be the main factor responsible for the development of ED in the systemic circulation. The systemic ED is manifested by an increased production of vasodilator molecules, mainly NO [46, 47], a vasodilator that is secreted by the endothelial and vascular smooth muscle cells [48] and that also has certain anti-inflammatory and antithrombotic properties [7]. The increased vasodilator tone in the systemic circulation leads to increased endothelial-dependent relaxation and increased blood flow, which consequently leads to the development of hyperdynamic circulation (HC) [49–51].

As a result of the vascular stress and increased concentration of some circulatory factors such as catecholamines, estrogens, and substance P that stimulate the endothelial synthetic activity [52, 53] several typical hemodynamic disorders occur in cirrhotic patients. The HC is one of the main and most typical hemodynamic features of patients with liver cirrhosis and PH [54–57]. It occurs as a result of a specific combination of several hemodynamic abnormalities, but the increased NO production is considered to be the major factor in the development of HC [54–57]. In this context, some studies have confirmed a significant correlation between the level of vWF and the NO production which may suggest a common activation mechanism [27]. HC is characterized by increased intrahepatic vascular resistance as a result of intrahepatic vasoconstriction and increased systemic vasodilation leading to an increased portal flow. The presence of HC in patients with liver cirrhosis is manifested by hypotension, low vascular resistance, and increased cardiac output, which develops as a compensation of the systemic vasodilation [9, 58]. Additionally, increased portal systemic shunting and reduced renal flow also occur [3, 59]. The severity of the HC has been significantly associated with the degree of PH, that is, by activating the NO synthetase, the portal pressure is an important factor that regulates the vasodilation in the splanchnic circulation [60]. Hence, in patients with liver cirrhosis, in addition to the endotoxemia, PH is thought to act as a factor of increased endothelial stress and stimulates additional NO production [52], i.e., the PH indirectly emphasizes the vasodilation in the splanchnic circulation.

4. Von-willebrand factor as an indicator of endothelial dysfunction and factor of PH progression

Some mediators secreted by the activated EC such as NO, vWF, P-selectin and Isoprostran are used as indicators of ED [26, 29, 61–63]. The important role of vWF in the process of angiogenesis, inflammation, cell proliferation and tumor growth has recently been increasingly emphasized [64]. Considering the fact that liver cirrhosis is closely related to ED, vWF as an indicator of ED causes considerable attention in cirrhotic patients. Since vWF is also involved in the pathogenesis and progression of PH, its value as a prognostic indicator in these patients becomes even more important.

vWF is a large multimeric glycoprotein released by the megakaryocytes and the activated vascular EC that plays a role in the process of primary hemostasis and coagulation [65]. In a coordinated manner, the function of vWF is regulated by two platelet membrane receptors, glycoprotein Ib (GPIb/IX/V) and glycoprotein IIb/IIIa [16, 66]. During primary hemostasis, vWF participates in both platelet adhesion and platelet aggregation. In case of endothelial damage, circulating vWF binds to exposed collagen in subendothelial structures and interacts with the platelet receptor GPIb/IX/V. This transient interaction enables subsequent stable interaction between platelets and collagen through the collagen receptor α2ß1 and glycoprotein VI [67]. This is followed by the exposure and activation of the receptor GP IIb/IIIa resulting in the release of platelet activating mediators such as *Adenosine diphosphate (A*DP) and TXA2. By binding to the GP IIb/IIIa receptor, the vWF participates in platelet aggregation and plug formation [16, 58]. Except in primary hemostasis, vWF also acts as a carrier of factor VIII protecting it from the proteolytic action of protein C and its cofactor protein S [68, 69].

Human EC has the capacity to synthesize vWF multimers with a higher molecular weight called ultra-large molecular weight multimers (ULMWM) [70]. After secretion by the EC, ULMWM usually undergo a process of fractionation to smaller vWF forms that are normally present in the circulation [70–72]. vWF is continuously secreted by the EC and megakaryocytes, while the ULMWM are stored in the cytoplasmic granules and are released after their degranulation as a response to a significant endothelial damage [73]. Contrary to the small vWG multimers, ULMWMs are the most haemostatically active forms of vWF that have the property of spontaneous binding to platelets and subendothelial structures, and are considered prothrombotic [74]. The multimeric composition of vWF is regulated by its protease ADAMTS13 [67], a clearance metalloprotease synthesized in hepatic stellate cells [75, 76] that processes ULMWM into smaller vWF forms [67, 75, 76]. The vWF activity is strictly regulated by ADAMTS13 and the vWF reactivity towards platelets is proportional to the size of the vWF multimers [9]. Since ADAMTS13 is synthesized in the liver [77], as expected, some studies have confirmed a markedly reduced concentration of ADAMTS13 in patients with liver disease [78]. In some patients Lisman et al. also confirmed reduced ADAMTS13 concentration, but in others the concentration and activity of ADAMTS13 has been elevated [67]. This may be due to its reduced clearance of ADAMTS13 or its reduced release from platelets [79] as a consequence of platelet activation secondary to disseminated intravascular coagulation (DIC). Although in advanced liver disease the synthesis function of the hepatocytes is generally reduced, the stellate cells tend to have an increased synthetic activity [80, 81] which may also explain the increased synthesis of ADAMTS13 registered in some patients.

It has been established that intrahepatic and systemic ED is involved in the pathogenesis and progression of PH. Since vWF is an indicator of ED, vWF recently has gained an important role as a prognostic indicator in cirrhotic patients. There are many mechanisms that are related to the increased vWF production in cirrhotic patients. The intrahepatic production of vWF as a result of the intrahepatic ED has been confirmed by the positive immune staining of vWF in sinusoidal endothelial cells in these patients [82, 83]. Also, the presence of endotoxemia and bacterial products, especially in advanced diseases appear to be the most important cause of increased endothelial secretion of vWF [58, 67], which has been confirmed by the linear increase in vWF concentration with the increase of endotoxemia [58, 84]. In addition to the increased endothelial production of vWF, there are other mechanisms that contribute to the increase in vWF such as increased shear stress, bacterial infections [58, 85], neoplastic processes, physical activity, or interferon-based therapy [86, 87]. Decreased expression or activity of ADAMTS13 recorded in some cirrhotic patients may also result in reduced clearance and increased vWF concentration [79]. It is also considered that increased vWF values may be related to the hyperfibrinolysis found in some patients, but on the other hand increased vWF has been also registered in patients without evidence of an increased proteolysis [58], which means that this is probably not a dominant mechanism.

Not only vWF is an indicator of ED, but the clinical and prognostic relevance of vWF is more pronounced because vWF is involved in the progression of PH. Since vWF is a large multimeric molecule, its increased concentration along with other abnormalities that favor procoagulant tendency in cirrhotic patients often results in occurrence of thrombosis in the hepatic microcirculation. If this is a long-term and continuous process, then it progressively obliterates and increases the resistance in the portal vasculature [67, 88] that leads to additional worsening of the PH. Additionally, it is assumed that when these thrombotic events are localized in the intestinal microcirculation they favor enterocytic ischemia and consequent intestinal bacterial translocation causing endotoxemia, which is crucial for the development of the majority of PH-related complications [9]. The literature data confirm a correlation between the concentration of vWF and the HVPG values [7, 16] suggesting that vWF level reflects the degree of PH. Also, vWF level has been related to some complications of PH such as hepatopulmonary syndrome and esopgaheal varices [89, 90].

The presence of PH is related to most of the complications in cirrhotic patients that define the course of the disease and more importantly the prognosis in these patients. Since vWF reflects PH, recent evidence emphasizes the importance of vWF as a predictor of mortality. Most studies that have analyzed the association between vWF and chronic liver disease have reported that vWF concentration correlates with the stage of liver disease assessed by Child-Turcotte-Pugh (CTP) and Model for End-Stage Liver Disease (MELD) score [7, 27, 91], that vWF can predict acute decompensation [16], occurrence of clinical events and PH-related complication [7, 92] and that vWF is an independent predictor of mortality that equals MELD score [7, 16, 91].

5. The relation between systemic inflammation and adverse outcomes in cirrhotic patients and the prognostic role of C-reactive protein

It has been established that systemic inflammation (SI) is common in patients with advanced liver disease and PH [93] and that the presence of SI in these patients has been associated with adverse outcomes [94–96] and a poor prognosis [95, 97–99]. The negative impact of SI on liver disease is reflected mainly through the increase in the portal pressure and in the reduction of the hepatic blood flow i.e. through deterioration of PH and liver disease progression [100].

SI is defined as a state of persistent and inadequate stimulation of the immune system, which is manifested by the presence of elevated inflammatory cytokines and activated immune cells [101]. The presence of SI is usually assessed by the presence of systemic inflammatory response syndrome (SIRS), a set of hemodynamic alteration that develops as a response to SI. The presence of SIRS is usually confirmed by specific diagnostic criteria. Sepsis is a condition of a systemic inflammatory response to infection, which involves a characteristic range of pathological changes in many host systems. The pathophysiological sequence involves release of cytokines and endothelial and neutrophil activation, which initiates a cascade of leukocyte-endothelial interaction and adhesion. This is followed by transendothelial migration and subsequent microvascular and tissue damage, consequently leading to a multiple organ failure [102]. It has been reported that endothelial and tissue damage correlates with the intensity of the inflammatory response and leukocyte sequestration in tissues [103].

It is known that SIRS most commonly develops in the context of acute bacterial infection. In patients with liver cirrhosis acute bacterial infection (respiratory, urinary etc.) can often cause an acute deterioration of liver function, which is mainly due to the effects of the SIRS. This may be a result of some specific features of the liver sinusoidal endothelial cells (SEC) that are not typical for the endothelial cells at other locations in the body. The liver SEC are fenestrated allowing inflammatory cells to pass through easily and come into direct contact with hepatocytes [104]. Additionally, the inflammatory cytokines within SI stimulate release of vWF from the EC [105, 106] and suppress the synthesis of ADAMTS13 in the stellate cells [105, 107] which may also contribute to the vWF rise and reflect the relation between SI and ED in cirrhotic patients. It has been also established that SI is underlying many of the PH-related complications and acute events in cirrhotic patients [93]. It is considered that in critically ill patients with liver cirrhosis, these acute events are better taken into account by the use of the general prognostic scores [Acute Physiology and Chronic Health Evaluation (APACHE) II, Sequential Organ Failure Assessment (SOFA), Simplified Acute Physiology Score (SAPS)], which provide better short-term mortality prediction than the prognostic scores specifically designed for patients with liver cirrhosis such as CTP and MELD score [9, 108]. On the other hand, some disorders related to liver disease, PH or HC may modify the clinical and biochemical parameters included in the SIRS scores which decreases their value as SIRS indicators [95]. Hypersplenism may mask leukocytosis or exacerbate leucopenia; subclinical encephalopathy may increase the respiratory rate and favor hypercapnia; hyperkinetic circulatory syndrome may increase the heart rate, and beta blockers may mask the tachycardia. This means that the presence of SIRS in patients with liver cirrhosis may often be underestimated by the scores and criteria for SIRS [93, 109]. Considering all the above, many researchers have focused on identifying new biological variables that would be more accurate indicators of SIRS than the currently used criteria. In this context, the value of serum C-reactive protein (CRP) as a surrogate marker of SIRS has recently been increasingly recognized [9].

CRP is an acute-phase inflammation protein that is synthesized in the liver mainly by interleukin 6. Moreover, it has been shown that CRP synthesis is preserved even in advanced liver disease [110, 111], which makes CRP a reliable SIRS indicator in this category of patients. Many researchers evaluated the predictive value of CRP in the general population and also in patients with liver cirrhosis. In the everyday clinical practice elevated CRP has been mainly used as an indicator of bacterial infection and many researchers have confirmed this relation [112–114]. Lazzarotto et al. defined that CRP value of 29.5 mg/L (sensitivity 82% and specificity 81%) is a reliable indicator of bacterial infection in cirrhotic patients [112]. Moreover, recent evidence suggests that the significant prognostic value of CRP in cirrhotic patients comes from the fact that in advanced liver cirrhosis, elevated CRP may persist after a bacterial infection has resolved [9] or it may also reflect the presence of a low grade SI that is not directly related to bacterial infection [108]. This is probably related to the endotoxemia and the bacterial products reaching systemic circulation.

The presence of SI in cirrhotic patients has the potential to trigger several serious complications and acute events related to PH and liver disease such as encephalopathy [68], renal failure [65, 70] or infection [108] and it has been related to negative outcomes during acute [115–117] or chronic [94–96] liver failure. Also, elevated CRP has been related to the organ failure and liver disease-related mortality [93, 112, 118]. Lazzarotto et al. confirmed that in patients with liver cirrhosis higher initial CRP values were associated with death before the ninetieth day of hospitalization [112]. Cervoni et al. demonstrated that mortality in liver cirrhosis was independently associated with CRP, MELD score, and extrahepatic comorbidities. They defined a CRP cut-off value of 29 mg/L persisting for 15 days after hospitalization to have the best sensitivity and specificity for predicting mortality in cirrhotic patients [93]. By using the variables found to be independent predictors of a six-month mortality (variations in CRP, MELD score and extrahepatic comorbidities) in the previous research [93], Di Martino et al. developed a prognostic model in order to predict the three-month mortality in patients with advanced liver cirrhosis and in a subgroup of patients with acute decompensation. They found that the MELD score [HR1.10; 95% CI, (1.05–1.14); $P < 0.001$] and mean CRP above 32 mg/L at baseline or 15 days after hospitalization [HR 2.21; 95% CI (1.03–4.76), $P = 0.042$) were independent predictors of the three-month mortality. Moreover, the study showed better diagnostic efficacy of the prognostic model than the diagnostic efficacy of the MELD score (AUROC, 0.789 vs. 0.734; $P = 0.043$) [118]. Also, a positive correlation was registered between CRP and MELD score in the whole population, but such correlation was not registered in the subgroup of patients with end-stage liver disease. These findings suggested that the presence of SI was clinically more significant in patients with advanced liver disease, that the prognostic significance of the CRP variations as indicators of SI was greater in more severe patients and that the presence of SI could not be adequately assessed by using the

MELD score. These findings once again emphasize the significant role of CRP as a prognostic indicator in patients with liver cirrhosis, especially in advanced disease.

6. The relation between endothelial dysfunction, systemic inflammation and haemostatic abnormalities in chronic liver disease

The haemostatic process is a strictly regulated system in which the process of conversion of fibrinogen into fibrin is consequently followed by its subsequent degradation [119]. Since most coagulation factors and fibrinolytic proteins are synthesized in the liver, a proper hepatic function is of particular importance for the perfectly synchronized function of the haemostatic process. Hence, acute and chronic liver conditions often have an intense influence on the process of hemostasis [120] and advanced liver disease is associated with many complex abnormalities in all three parts of the haemostatic process. In patients with liver cirrhosis the haemostatic dysfunction is related to several mechanisms, such as quantitative and qualitative platelet abnormalities, quantitative and qualitative abnormalities in the coagulation factors and fibrinolytic proteins, reduced clearance of activated coagulation factors, abnormalities in the process of fibrinolysis, as well as to the presence of intensified fibrinolysis and low grade intravascular coagulation [121–123].

The primary hemostasis reflects the interaction between the platelets and the blood vessel and it is mediated by the action of vWF. Thrombocytopenia and the variable thrombocytopathy are the two most common abnormalities in cirrhotic patients within the primary hemostasis [124]. Thrombocytopenia occurs as a result of the increased sequestration due to splenomegaly, decreased thrombopoietin level and myelosuppression, increased systemic immune activation due to portosystemic shunting, impaired intestinal barrier and increased endotoxemia, immune-mediated platelet destruction and due to the platelet consumption within low grade intravascular coagulation [125–129]. The platelet dysfunction is presented as a reduced transmembrane signaling and progressive inability for platelet activation as a response to several stimuli such as adenosine diphosphate, thrombin, collagen, epinephrine or rhizocetine. This dysfunction results in insufficient production of thromboxane and serotonin and precipitates cascade abnormalities in the process of platelet aggregation [130, 131].

The central part of the haemostatic process is the process of coagulation, also called secondary homeostasis or thrombin generation. Most coagulation factors, such as fibrinogen, factor V, VII, VIII, IX, X, XI, XII are synthesized in the liver, which means if the liver synthetic function is impaired, their level inevitably decreases [132]. On the other hand, in patients with liver cirrhosis the synthesis of the anticoagulant proteins, such as protein C, protein S, and antithrombin is also reduced which partially compensate for the procoagulant deficiency. Despite the decreased concentration of most coagulation factors, in cirrhotic patients there is an increased concentration of factor VIII and vWF, two coagulation factors that are considered acute phase reactants [133–137]. Due to the reduced synthesis of the coagulation factors of the external pathway (mainly factor VII) prolonged prothrombin time (PT) is usually registered, while the reduced synthesis of the coagulation factors of the internal pathway results in prolongation of the activated partial thromboplastin time (aPTT). Thrombin time (TT) reflects the final step of the coagulation cascade, the conversion of fibrinogen into fibrin. TT reflects quantitative and qualitative fibrinogen abnormalities, a state called dysfibrinogenemia. Fibrinogen is also an acute phase reactant and in patients with mild or moderate liver cirrhosis it can be normal or slightly elevated [138, 139]. On the contrary, in advanced, severe cirrhosis fibrinogen concentration is usually decreased [139] resulting in prolongation of the TT. Fibrinogen is almost exclusively synthesized in the liver and hypofibrinogenemia in these patients could be a consequence of the reduced synthetic liver capacity, the increased metabolism, the abnormal fibrinolytic activity or the consumption as part of the DIC [140].

The final phase of the haemostatic process is fibrinolysis, the process of thrombus dissolution that limits the coagulation cascade. The fibrinolytic impulse is generated by the tissue plasminogen activator (t-PA), uricinase plasminogen activator and activated factor XII. They induce the conversion of plasminogen to plasmin, which then acts on fibrin to produce the fibrin degradation products (FDP). Deviations in the fibrinolysis in cirrhotic patients occur as a result of the decreased hepatocyte function, vitamin K deficiency and presence of hyperfibrinolysis [48, 141] which has been registered in about one third of the cirrhotic patients [48, 142–144]. The presence of hyperfibrinolysis and DIC in patients with liver cirrhosis is still the subject of a wide debate [145]. According to some studies, the abnormalities in the hyperfibrinolitic process correlate with the CTP score and are more prevalent in the elderly and in patients with decompensated cirrhosis [146, 147]. Primary hyperfibrinolysis occurs due to the increased concentration of t-PA (as a consequence of impaired hepatic clearance) and decreased concentration or functionality of antiplasmin and other plasminogen activator inhibitors [148–151], which leads to an increased conversion of plasminogen to plasmin [152]. The secondary hyperfibrinolysis develops as a continuum of an emphasized coagulation, most commonly within DIC. Although DIC has been registered in a small number of patients with hyperfibrinolysis, it rarely has a significant clinical impact [152].

An important perspective of the hyperfibrinolysis in cirrhotic patients is its relation to the increased bleeding risk and to the increased incidence of portal vein thrombosis (PVT). FDP created during hyperfibrinolysis interfere with the process of fibrin polymerization by inhibiting the platelet aggregation and thus increasing the risk of bleeding. As the measurement of individual components of the fibrinolytic pathway is of little use in the assessment of this tendency, the role of hyperfibrinolysis in the pathogenesis of bleeding in patients with liver cirrhosis is still not completely clear [142]. On the other hand, the relation between elevated D-dimers and PVT in cirrhotic patients has also been evaluated. Most studies that analyzed the relation and prognostic role of D-dimers in these patients confirmed significant association between the elevated D-dimers and the occurrence of PVT [153, 154]. One study suggested that the risk of developing PVT in patients with liver cirrhosis was significantly higher in case of a significant postoperative rise in the D-dimers concentration that exceeded 16,000 ng/ml [153]. Zhang et al. confirmed significant association between the elevated D-dimers and the occurrence of PVT independent of the CTP score [154]. Additionally, a meta-analysis of 21 studies found that increased concentration of D-dimers was associated with an increased risk of PVT not related to surgery, suggesting that D-dimers could be used as a diagnostic marker for PVT in cirrhotic patients [155]. However, not all studies confirmed this relation. A retrospective observational study of 66 patients did not find any significant difference in the D-dimers level between cirrhotic patients with and without PVT [156]. Most studies suggest that elevated D-dimers in cirrhotic patients correlate with the degree of liver dysfunction which is probably related to the increased hyperfibrinolysis in advanced liver disease [144, 157, 158]. More importantly, it has also been established that in patients with liver cirrhosis elevated D-dimers were related to poor outcomes [144, 154, 157, 158] and that they were significant predictor of short-term mortality [157, 158]. These findings suggest that in critically ill cirrhotic patients or in some specific clinical settings monitoring of the D-dimers concentration may have some useful clinical and prognostic implication.

It is well established that the significantly reduced synthetic liver function in advanced disease is responsible for the reduced synthesis of the coagulation factors. But, since this occurs late in the stage of the disease, several other mechanisms might be responsible for many complex abnormalities in the coagulation process in cirrhotic patients. In this context, the ED in patients with liver cirrhosis seems to be largely involved in this process through several mechanisms [48]. The process of ED by itself among other disturbances implies an imbalance in the secretion of pro-coagulants, anticoagulants, and also fibrinolytic substances, which can be responsible for some of the haemostatic abnormalities. Also, some evidence suggests that in patients with liver cirrhosis there is a direct relation between the endotoxemia and coagulation activity i.e. that endotoxemia can directly activates the coagulation and fibrinolytic pathway in patients with liver cirrhosis [159]. In this context, some researchers have demonstrated a strong association between endotoxemia and high levels of prothrombin fragments F1 + 2, which are markers of thrombin generation [159, 160], and also between endotoxemia and elevated D-dimers, which are markers of hyperfibrinolysis [159]. This is confirmed by the fact that in cirrhotic patients with elevated F1 + 2 and D-dimers a reduction in the coagulation and fibrinolytic activity has been registered after reduction of endotoxemia [159]. Some data also confirm a direct association between endotoxin and a thrombin-antithrombin complex [160]. Endothelial activation may also explain the relationship between the synchronized rise of vWF and D-dimers as part of secondary hyperfibrinolysis. Lisman et al. extensively analyzed the qualitative and quantitative deviations of vWF in patients with liver cirrhosis and found elevated levels of propeptide indicating an acute endothelial damage, presumably associated to the presence of low grade DIC [67]. It is considered that the increased plasma proteolysis in these patients leads to increased concentrations of vWF as well as highly reactive vWF multimers [161, 162]. The endotoxin also has a potential to induce increased expression of tissue factor (TF) on the surface of the macrophages and to stimulate synthesis of tumor necrotic factor (TNF), which activates the external coagulation pathway [118, 163–165]. The presence of SI in cirrhotic patients also has an influence on the coagulation process. In terms of severe inflammation, the inflammatory cytokines activate the endothelial cells, inhibit the liver synthesis of protein C [166] and can stimulate degranulation of the cytoplasmic granules and release of ULMWM [105, 107], the most prothrombotic vWF multimers. Among other complex haemostatic abnormalities in cirrhotic patients, the increased concentration of ULMWM confirmed in some patients with acute decompensation [167] is considered to be related to the increased prothrombotic tendency.

7. Conclusion

All the above suggests a close relation between SI, ED, and liver disease-related coagulopathy in cirrhotic patients and emphasizes their important role in the pathogenesis of majority of manifestations and complications of PH. It also explains the crucial role of endotoxemia as a central initiating factor in their pathogenesis. Elevated vWF reflecting ED and significant and prolonged CRP rise reflecting SI should be routinely used in the everyday clinical practice. Additional research is needed in order to insert more deeply into the patogenesis of these entities and to propose new variables that would reflect their presence and significance more precisely.

Conflict of interest

The author declares no conflict of interest.

Author details

Elena Curakova Ristovska[1,2]*

1 University Clinic for Gastroenterohepatology, Skopje, Republic of North Macedonia

2 Faculty of Medicine, Ss. Cyril and Methodius University in Skopje, Skopje, Republic of North Macedonia

*Address all correspondence to: elenacurakova@yahoo.com

References

[1] D'Amico G, Garcia-Tsao G, Pagliaro L. Natural history and prognostic indicators of survival in cirrhosis:a systematic review of 118 studies. J Hepatol. 2006;44(1):217-231.

[2] Kamegaya K. Definition and classification of liver cirrhosis. Nihon Rinsho. 1994 Jan;52(1):11-8. Japanese. PMID: 8114278.

[3] Bosch J, Garcia-Pagan JC. Complications of cirrhosis. I. Portal hypertension. J Hepatol 2000;32(1 Suppl):141-56.

[4] Iwakiri Y, Groszmann RJ. Vascular endothelial dysfunction in cirrhosis. J Hepatol 2007;46:927-934.

[5] Matei V, Rodriguez-Vilarrupla A, Deulofeu R, et al. The eNOS cofactor tetrahydrobiopterin improves endothelial dysfunction in livers of rats with CCl4 cirrhosis. Hepatology 2006;44:44-52.

[6] Gracia-Sancho J, Lavina B, Rodriguez-Vilarrupla A, et al. Increased oxidative stress in cirrhotic rat livers: a potential mechanism contributing to reduced nitric oxide bioavailability. Hepatology 2008;47:1248-56.

[7] La Mura V, Reverter JC, Flores-Arroyo A, Raffa S, Reverter E, Seijo S, et al. Von Willebrand factor levels predict clinical outcome in patients with cirrhosis and portal hypertension. Gut 2011;60:1133-1138

[8] Tripodi A. Liver Disease and Hemostatic (Dys)function. Semin Thromb Hemost. 2015; 41(5):462-7

[9] Di Martino V, Weil D, Cervoni JP, Thevenot T. New prognostic markers in liver cirrhosis. World J Hepatol. 2015 May 28;7(9):1244-50.

[10] Bosch J, Abraldes JG, Berzigotti A, Garcia-Pagan JC. The clinical use of HVPG measurements in chronic liver disease. Nature reviews Gastroenterology & hepatology. 2009; 6(10):573-82.

[11] Hametner S, Ferlitsch A, Ferlitsch M, et al. The VITRO Score (Von Willebrand Factor Antigen/ Thrombocyte Ratio) as a New Marker for Clinically Significant Portal Hypertension in Comparison to Other Non-Invasive Parameters of Fibrosis Including ELF Test. PLoS One. 2016;11(2):e0149230..

[12] Bosch J, Garcia-Pagan JC, Berzigotti A, Abraldes JG. Measurement of portal pressure and its role in the management of chronic liver disease. Seminars in liver disease. 2006; 26(4):348-62. Epub 2006/10/20.

[13] de Franchis R. Revising consensus in portal hypertension: report of the Baveno V consensus workshop on methodology of diagnosis and therapy in portal hypertension. J Hepatol 2010; 53 (4):762-8.

[14] Ripoll C, Groszmann RJ, Garcia-Tsao G, Bosch J, Grace N, Burroughs A, et al. Hepatic venous pressure gradient predicts development of hepatocellular carcinoma independently of severity of cirrhosis. J Hepatol 2009; 50(5):923-8.

[15] Peck-Radosavljevic M, Angermayr B, Datz C, Ferlitsch A, Ferlitsch M, Fuhrmann V, et al. Austrian consensus on the definition and treatment of portal hypertension and its complications (Billroth II). Wieneklinische Wochenschrift. 2013; 125(7-8):200-19

[16] Ferlitsch M, Reiberger T, Hoke M, SalzlP,SchwengererB,UlbrichG,PayerBA, Trauner M, Peck-Radosavljevic M, Ferlitsch A. von Willebrand factor as new noninvasive predictor of portal

hypertension, decompensation and mortality in patients with liver cirrhosis. Hepatology 2012; 56: 1439-1447

[17] Reiberger T, Ferlitsch A, Payer BA, Pinter M, Homoncik M, Peck-Radosavljevic M. Non-selective beta-blockers improve the correlation of liver stiffness and portal pressure in advanced cirrhosis. Journal of gastroenterology. 2012; 47(5):561-8.

[18] dc Franchis R. Expanding consensus in portal hypertension: Report of the Baveno VI Consensus Workshop: Stratifying risk and individualizing care for portal hypertension. J Hepatol 2015.

[19] D'Amico G, Morabito A, Pagliaro L, Marubini E. Survival and prognostic indicators in compensated and decompensated cirrhosis. Dig Dis Sci 1986;31:468-475

[20] D'Amico G, Pasta L, Madonia S, Tarantino G, Mancuso A, Malizia G, et al. The incidence of esophageal varices in cirrhosis. Gastroenterology 2001;120:A2.

[21] D'Amico G. Natural history of compensated cirrhosis and varices. In: Boyer TD, Groszmann RJ, editors. Complications of cirrhosis: pathogenesis, consequences and therapy. American Association for the Study of Liver Diseases; 2001. p. 118-123

[22] Samonakis DN, Koulentaki M, Coucoutsi C, et al. Clinical outcomes of compensated and decompensated cirrhosis: A long term study. World J Hepatol. 2014;6(7):504-512.

[23] D'Amico G, Garcia–Tsao G, Abraldes J, Gine's P, Kim WR, Schepis F, et al. Prognostic indicators in cirrhosis. In: de Franchis R, editor. Portal Hypertension IV. Proceedings of the Fourth Baveno International Consensus Workshop on Definitions, Methodology and Therapeutic Strategies. Blackwell, 2005

[24] Cabre E, Abad-Lacruz A, Nunez MC, Gonzalez-Huix F, Fernandez- Banares F, Gil A, et al. The relationship of plasma polyunsaturated fatty acid deficiency with survival in advanced liver cirrhosis: multivariate analysis. Am J Gastroenterol 1993;88:718-722

[25] Caballero AE. Endothelial dysfunction in obesity and insulin resistance: a road to diabetes and heart disease. Obes Res 2003;11:1278-1289

[26] van Mourik JA, Boertjes R, Huisveld IA, et al. von Willebrand factor propeptide in vascular disorders: A tool to distinguish between acute and chronic endothelial cell perturbation. Blood. 1999;94(1):179-185.

[27] Albornoz L, Alvarez D, Otaso JC, et al. Von Willebrand factor could be an index of endothelial dysfunction in patients with cirrhosis: relationship to degree of liver failure and nitric oxide levels. J Hepatol 1999;30:451-5

[28] Blann A. Von Willebrand factor and the endothelium in vascular disease. Br J Biomed Sci 1993;50:125-134.

[29] Spiel AO, Gilbert JC, Jilma B. Von Willebrand factor in cardiovascular disease: focus on acute coronary syndromes. Circulation 2008;117:1449-1459.

[30] Lip GY, Blann A. Von Willebrand factor: a marker of endothelial dysfunction in vascular disorders? Cardiovasc Res 1997;34:255-265.

[31] Szmitko PE, Wang CH, Weisel RD, de Almeida JR, Anderson TJ, Verma S. New markers of inflammation and endothelial cell activation: part I. Circulation 2003;108:1917-1923.

[32] Budhiraja R, Tuder RM, Hassoun PM. Endothelial dysfunction in pulmonary hypertension. Circulation 2004;109:159-165

[33] Albillos A, Hera Ad Ade L, Reyes E, Monserrat J, Munoz L, Nieto M, et al. Tumour necrosis factor-alpha expression by activated monocytes and altered T-cell homeostasis in ascitic alcoholic cirrhosis: amelioration with norfloxacin. J Hepatol 2004;40:624-631.

[34] Genesca J, Marti R, Gonzalez A, Torregrosa M, Segura R. Soluble interleukin- 6 receptor levels in liver cirrhosis. Am J Gastroenterol 1999;94:3074-3075.

[35] Lopez-Talavera JC, Levitzki A, Martinez M, Gazit A, Esteban R, Guardia J. Tyrosine kinase inhibition ameliorates the hyperdynamic state and decreases nitric oxide production in cirrhotic rats with portal hypertension and ascites. J Clin Invest 1997;100:664-670.

[36] Giron-GonzalezJA,Martinez-SierraC, Rodriguez-Ramos C, Rendon P, Macias MA, Fernandez-Gutierrez C, et al. Adhesion molecules as a prognostic marker of liver cirrhosis. Scand J Gastroenterol 2005;40: 217-224.

[37] Buck M, Garcia-Tsao G, Groszmann RJ, Stalling C, Grace ND, Burroughs AK, et al. Novel inflammatory biomarkers of portal pressure in compensated cirrhosis patients. Hepatology 2014;59:1052-1059

[38] Wiese S, Mortensen C, Gotze JP, Christensen E, Andersen O, Bendtsen F, et al. Cardiac and proinflammatory markers predict prognosis in cirrhosis. Liver Int 2013;34:e19-30.

[39] Guarner C, Soriano G, Tomas A, Bulbena O, Novella MT, Balanzo J, et al. Increased serum nitrite and nitrate levels in patients with cirrhosis: relationship to endotoxemia. Hepatology 1993;18:1139-1143.

[40] Campillo B, Bories PN, Benvenuti C, Dupeyron C. Serum and urinary nitrate levels in liver cirrhosis: endotoxemia, renal function and hyperdynamic circulation. J Hepatol 1996;25:707-714.

[41] Tazi KA, Moreau R, Herve P, Dauvergne A, Cazals-Hatem D, Bert F, et al. Norfloxacin reduces aortic NO synthases and proinflammatory cytokine up- regulation in cirrhotic rats: role of Akt signaling. Gastroenterology 2005;129:303-314.

[42] Bellis L, Berzigotti A, Abraldes JG, Moitinho E, Garcia-Pagan JC, Bosch J, et al. Low doses of isosorbide mononitrate attenuate the postprandial increase in portal pressure in patients with cirrhosis. Hepatology 2003;37:378-384

[43] Groszmann RJ, Abraldes JG. Portal hypertension: from bedside to bench. J Clin Gastroenterol 2005;39:S125–S130.

[44] Wiest R, Groszmann RJ. The paradox of nitric oxide in cirrhosis and portal hypertension: too much, not enough. Hepatology 2002;35:478-491.

[45] Groszmann RJ, Loureiro-Silva M, Tsai MH. The biology of portal hypertension. 4 ed. New York: Lippincott Williams and Wilkins; 2001, 679-97.

[46] Vallance P, Moncada S. Hyperdynamic circulation in cirrhosis: a role for nitric oxide. Lancet 1991;337:776-778.

[47] Bomzon A, Blendis LM. The nitric oxide hypothesis and the hyperdynamic circulation in cirrhosis. Hepatology 1994;20:1343-1350

[48] Ferro D, Quintarelli C, Saliola M, Alessandri C, Basili S, Bonavita MS, Violi F. Prevalence of hyperfibrinolysis in patients with liver cirrhosis. Fibrinolysis 1993;7:59-62

[49] Shah V, Toruner M, Haddad F, Cadelina G, Papapetropoulos A, Choo K, Sessa WC, Groszmann RJ.

Impaired endothelial nitric oxide synthase activity associated with enhanced caveolin binding in experimental cirrhosis in the rat. Gastroenterology 1999; 117: 1222-1228

[50] Tsai MH, Iwakiri Y, Cadelina G, Sessa WC, Groszmann RJ. Mesenteric vasoconstriction triggers nitric oxide overproduction in the superior mesenteric artery of portal hypertensive rats. Gastroenterology 2003;125:1452-1461.

[51] Wiest R, Shah V, Sessa WC, Groszmann RJ. NO overproduction by eNOS precedes hyperdynamic splanchnic circulation in portal hypertensive rats. Am J Physiol 1999;276:G1043–G1051.

[52] Sterling R, Sanyal A, Schubert M. Nitric oxide and portal hypertension Gastroenterology, 112 (1997), pp. 1767-1768

[53] Blann AD, Naqvi T, Waite M, McCollum CN. Von Willebrand factor and endothelial damage in essential hypertension o J Hum Hypertens, 7 (1993), pp. 107-111

[54] Pizcucta MP, Piqué JM, Bosch J, Whittle BJR, Moncada S. Effeets of inhibiting nitric oxide biosynthesis on the systemic and splanchnic circulation of rats with portal hypertension. Br J Pharmacol, 105 (1992), pp. 184-190

[55] Claria J, Jiménez W, Ros J, Rigol M, Angeli P, Arroyo V, et al. Increased nitric oxide-dependent vasorelaxation in aortic rings of cirrhotic rats with ascites. Hepatology, 20 (1994), pp. 1615-1621.

[56] Sieber CC, Groszmann RJ. Nitric oxide mediates in vitro hyporeactivity to vasopressors in mesenteric vessels of portal hypertensive rats Gastroenterology, 103 (1992), pp. 235-239.

[57] Castro A, Jiménez W, Claria J, Ros J, Martinez JM, Bosch M, et al. Impaired responsiveness to angiotensin II in experimental cirrhosis: role of nitric oxide. Hepatology, 18 (1993), pp. 367-372.

[58] Ferro D, Quintarelli C, Lattuada A, Leo R, Alessandroni M, Mannucci PM, et al. High plasma levels of von Willebrand factor as a marker of endothelial perturbation in cirrhosis: relationship to endotoxemia. Hepatology 1996;23:1377-1383

[59] Newby DE, Jalan R, Masumori S, Hayes PC, Boon NA, Webb DJ. Peripheral vascular tone in patients with cirrhosis: role of the renin-angiotensin and sympathetic nervous systems. Cardiovasc Res 1998;38:221-228.

[60] Abraldes JG, Iwakiri Y, Loureiro-Silva M, Haq O, Sessa WC, Groszmann RJ. Mild increases in portal pressure upregulate vascular endothelial growth factor and endothelial nitric oxide synthase in the intestinal microcirculatory bed, leading to a hyperdynamic state. Am J Physiol Gastrointest Liver Physiol 2006;290:G980–G987.

[61] Leon DA, McCambridge J. Liver cirrhosis mortality rates in Britain from 1950 to 2002: an analysis of routine data. Lancet 2006;367:52-6

[62] Smyth SS, McEver RP, Weyrich AS, et al. Platelet functions beyond hemostasis. J Thromb Haemost 2009;7:1759-66.

[63] Lavi S, Yang EH, Prasad A, et al. The interaction between coronary endothelial dysfunction, local oxidative stress, and endogenous nitric oxide in humans. Hypertension 2008;51:127-33.

[64] Lenting PJ, Casari C, Christophe OD, Denis CV (2012) von Willebrand factor: the old, the new and

the unknown. J Thromb Haemost 10: 2428-2437.

[65] Maieron A, Salzl P, Peck-Radosavljevic M, et al. Von Willebrand Factor as a new marker for non-invasive assessment of liver fibrosis and cirrhosis in patients with chronic hepatitis C. Aliment Pharmacol Ther. 2014;39(3):331-338

[66] Iannacone M, Sitia G, Isogawa M, et al. Platelets mediate cytotoxic T lymphocyte-induced liver damage. Nat Med 2005; 11: 1167-9

[67] Lisman T, Bongers TN, Adelmeijer J, et al. Elevated levels of von Willebrand Factor in cirrhosis support platelet adhesion despite reduced functional capacity. Hepatology. 2006;44(1):53-61

[68] Brinkhous KM, Sandberg H, Garris JB, et al. Purified human factor VIII procoagulant protein: comparative hemostatic response after infusions into hemophilic and von Willebrand disease dogs. Proc Natl Acad Sci U S A 1985; 82:8752.

[69] De Meyer SF, Deckmyn H, Vanhoorelbeke K. von Willebrand factor to the rescue. Blood 2009; 113:5049.

[70] Moake, J. L., C. K. Rudy, J. H. Troll, M. J. Weinstein, N. M. Colannino, J. Azocar, R. H. Seder, S. L. Hong, and D. Deykin. 1982. Unusually large plasma factor VIII: von Willebrand factor multimers in chronic relapsing thrombotic thrombocytopenic purpura. New Engl. J. Med. 307:1432-1435.

[71] Moake, J. L., J. J. Byrnes, J. H. Troll, C. K. Rudy, S. L. Hong, M. J. Weinstein, and N. M. Colannino. 1985. Effects of fresh frozen plasma and its cryosupernatant fraction on von Willebrand factor multimer forms in chronic relapsing thrombotic thrombocytopenic purpura. Blood. 65:1232-1236.

[72] Frangos, J., J. L. Moake, L. Nolasco, and L. McIntire. 1986. Evidence for an unusually large factor VIII: vWF depolymerase in normal plasma cryosupernatant. Clin. Res. 34:656A.

[73] Moake JL, Turner NA, Stathopoulos NA, Nolasco LH, Hellums JD. Involvement of large plasma von Willebrand factor (vWF) multimers and unusually large vWF forms derived from endothelial cells in shear stress-induced platelet aggregation. J Clin Invest. 1986;78(6):1456-1461

[74] Chow TW, Turner NA, Chintagumpala M, et al. Increased von Willebrand factor binding to platelets in single episode and recurrent types of thrombotic thrombocytopenic purpura. Am J Hematol 1998; 57:293.

[75] Zhou W, Inada M, Lee TP, et al. ADAMTS13 is expressed in hepatic stellate cells. Lab Invest 2005;85(06):780-788

[76] Uemura M, Tatsumi K, Matsumoto M, et al. Localization of ADAMTS13 to the stellate cells of human liver. Blood 2005;106 (03):922-924

[77] Zheng X, Chung D, Takayama TK, Majerus EM, Sadler JE, Fujikawa K. Structure of von Willebrand factor-cleaving protease (ADAMTS13), a metalloprotease involved in thrombotic thrombocytopenic purpura. J Biol Chem 2001; 276: 41059-41063.

[78] Mannucci PM, Canciani MT, Forza I, Lussana F, Lattuada A, Rossi E. Changes in health and disease of the metalloprotease that cleaves von Willebrand factor. Blood 2001;98(09):2730-2735

[79] Suzuki M, Murata M, Matsubara Y, Uchida T, Ishihara H, Shibano T, et al. Detection of von Willebrand factor-cleaving protease (ADAMTS13) in

human platelets. Biochem Biophys Res Commun 2004;313: 212-216

[80] Bataller R, Brenner DA. Liver fibrosis. J Clin Invest 2005;115:209-218.

[81] Atzori L, Poli G, Perra A. Hepatic stellate cell: a star cell in the liver. Int J Biochem Cell Biol 2009;41(8-9):1639-1642

[82] Knittel T, Neubauer K, Armbrust T, Ramadori G. Expression of von Willebrand factor in normal and diseased rat livers and in cultivated liver cells. Hepatology 1995;21:470-476.

[83] Wu H, Yan S, Wang G, Cui S, Zhang C, Zhu Q. Von Willebrand factor as a novel noninvasive predictor of portal hypertension and esophageal varices in hepatitis B patients with cirrhosis. Scand J Gastroenterol 2015;16:1-10

[84] Yilmaz VT, Dincer D, Avci AB, Cetinkaya R. Significant Association between Serum Levels of Von Willebrand Factor (vWF) Antigen with Stages of Cirrhosis. Eurasian J Med. 2015;47(1):21-25

[85] Gulley D, Teal E, Suvannasanka A, Chalasani N, Liangpusankul S. Deep vein thrombosis and pulmonary embolism in cirrhosis patients. Dig Dis Sci 2008;53:3012-3017

[86] Pramhas S, Homoncik M, Ferenci P, Ferlitsch A, Scherzer T, Gangl A, et al. von Willebrand factor antigen: a novel on-treatment predictor of response to antiviral therapy in chronic hepatitis C genotypes 1 and 4. Antiviral therapy. 2010; 15(6):831-9.

[87] Homoncik M, Ferlitsch A, Ferenci P, Formann E, Jilma B, Gangl A, et al. Short- and long-term effects of therapy with interferon-alpha and pegylated interferon-alpha/ribavirin on platelet plug formation and von Willebrand factor release in patients with chronic hepatitis C. Alimentary pharmacology & therapeutics. 2005; 21(1):49-55.

[88] Wannhoff A, Müller OJ, Friedrich K, et al. Effects of increased von Willebrand factor levels on primary hemostasis in thrombocytopenic patients with liver cirrhosis. PLoS One. 2014;9(11):e112583. Published 2014 Nov 14.

[89] Horvatits T, Drolz A, Roedl K, Herkner H, Ferlitsch A, Perkmann T, Müller C, Trauner M, Schenk P, Fuhrmann V. Von Willebrand factor antigen for detection of hepatopulmonary sundrome in patients with cirrhosis. J Hepatol. 2014 Sep;61(3):544-9.

[90] Mahmoud HS, Ghweil AA, Bazeed SE, Fayed HM, Meguid MMA: Reliability of Plasma Von Willebrand Factor Antigen in Prediction of Esophageal Varices in Patients with Liver Cirrhosis. Open Journal of Gastroenterology, 2015; 5, 49-57.

[91] Curakova Ristovska E, Genadieva-Dimitrova M, Caloska-Ivanova V, Misevski J. Von-Willebrand factor as a predictor of three-month mortality in patients with liver cirrhosis compared to MELD score. Acta Gastroenterol Belg. 2019 Oct-Dec;82(4):487-493. PMID: 31950803.

[92] Kalambokis GN, Oikonomou A, Christou L, et al. von Willebrand factor and procoagulant imbalance predict outcome in patients with cirrhosis and thrombocytopenia. J Hepatol. 2016;65(5):921-928.

[93] Cervoni JP, Thévenot T, Weil D, Muel E, Barbot O, Sheppard F, Monnet E, Di Martino V. C-reactive protein predicts short-term mortality in patients with cirrhosis. J Hepatol 2012; 56: 1299-1304

[94] Shawcross DL, Davies NA, Williams R, Jalan R. Systemic inflammatory response exacerbates the neuropsychological effects of induced hyperammonemia in cirrhosis. J Hepatol 2004;40:247-254.

[95] Cazzaniga M, Dionigi E, Gobbo G, Fioretti A, Monti V, Salerno F. The systemic inflammatory response syndrome in cirrhotic patients: relationship with their in-hospital outcome. J Hepatol 2009;51:475-482.

[96] Thabut D, Massard J, Gangloff A, Carbonell N, Francoz C, Nguyen-Khac E, et al. Model for end-stage liver disease score and systemic inflammatory response are major prognostic factors in patients with cirrhosis and acute functional renal failure. Hepatology 2007;46:1872-1882

[97] Dirchwolf M, Ruf AE. Role of systemic inflammation in cirrhosis: From pathogenesis to prognosis. World J Hepatol. 2015 Aug 8;7(16):1974-81.

[98] Abdel-Khalek EE, El-Fakhry A, Helaly M, Hamed M, Elbaz O. Systemic inflammatory response syndrome in patients with liver cirrhosis. Arab J Gastroenterol 2011; 12: 173-177.

[99] Behroozian R, Bayazidchi M, Rasooli J. Systemic Inflammatory Response Syndrome and MELD Score in Hospital Outcome of Patients with Liver Cirrhosis. Middle East J Dig Dis 2012; 4: 168-172.

[100] Jalan R, MookerjeeR. Systemic hemodynamic, hepatic blood flow and portal pressure in patients with cirrhosis and multiorgan failure: the role of sympathetic activation. Hepatology 2008: 48:1077A

[101] Albillos A, Lario M, Alvarez-Mon M. Cirrhosis-associated immune dysfunction: Distinct features and clinical relevance. J Hepatol 2014;61: 1385-1396

[102] Parrillo, J. E. 1993. Pathogenetic mechanisms of septic shock. N. Engl. J. Med. 328:1471-1477.

[103] Weiss, S. J. 1989. Tissue destruction by neutrophils. N. Engl. J. Med. 320:365-376.

[104] Braet F, Wisse E. Structural and functional aspects of liver sinusoidal endothelial cell fenestrae: a review. Comp Hepatol 2002;1:1.

[105] Bernardo A, Ball C, Nolasco L, Moake JF, Dong JF. Effects of inflammatory cytokines on the release and cleavage of the endothelial cell-derived ultra large vWF multimers under flow. Blood 2004;104: 100-106.

[106] Schorer AE, Moldow CF, Rick ME. Interleukin 1 or endotoxin increases the release of von Willebrand factor from human endothelial cells. Br J Haematol 1987;67:193-197.

[107] Cao WJ, Niiya M, Zheng XW, Shang DZ, Zheng XL. Inflammatory cytokines inhibit ADAMTS13 synthesis in hepatic stellate cells and endothelial cells. J Thromb Haemost 2008;6:1233-1235.

[108] Malik R, Mookerjee RP, Jalan R. Infection and inflammation in liver failure: two sides of the same coin. J Hepatol 2009;51:426-429.

[109] Curakova Ristovska E, Genadieva-Dimitrova M, Caloska-Ivanova V, Nikolovska E, Joksimovic N, Todorovska B, Isahi U, Milichevik I. The SIRS score relevance for assessment of systemic inflammation compared to C-reactive protein in patients with liver cirrhosis. *Macedonian Medical Review.* 2019; 73(1): 24-30

[110] Bota DP, Van Nuffelen M, Zakariah AN, Vincent JL. Serum levels of C-reactive protein and procalcitonin in critically ill patients with cirrhosis

of the liver. J Lab Clin Med 2005; 146: 347-351

[111] Park WB, Lee KD, Lee CS, Jang HC, Kim HB, Lee HS, Oh MD, Choe KW. Production of C-reactive protein in Escherichia coli-infected patients with liver dysfunction due to liver cirrhosis. Diagn Microbiol Infect Dis 2005; 51: 227-230

[112] Lazzarotto C, Ronsoni MF, Fayad L, et al. Acute phase proteins for the diagnosis of bacterial infection and prediction of mortality in acute complications of cirrhosis. Ann Hepatol. 2013;12(4):599-607.

[113] Papp M, Vitalis Z, Altorjay I, Tornai I, Udvardy M, Harsfalvi J, Vida A, et al. Acute phase proteins in the diagnosis and prediction of cirrhosis associated bacterial infections. Liver Int 2012; 32: 603-11.

[114] Tsiakalos A, Karatzaferis A, Ziakas P, Hatzis G. Acute- phase proteins as indicators of bacterial infection in patients with cirrhosis. Liver Int 2009; 29: 1538-42.

[115] Leithead JA, Ferguson JW, Bates CM, Davidson JS, Lee A, Bathgate AJ, et al. The systemic inflammatory response syndrome is predictive of renal dysfunction in patients with non-paracetamol-induced acute liver failure. Gut 2009;58:443-449.

[116] Rolando N, Wade J, Davalos M, Wendon J, Philpott-Howard J, Williams R. The systemic inflammatory response syndrome in acute liver failure. Hepatology 2000;32:734-739.

[117] Vaquero J, Polson J, Chung C, Helenowski I, Schiodt FV, Reisch J, et al. Infection and the progression of hepatic encephalopathy in acute liver failure. Gastroenterology 2003;125:755-764.

[118] Di Martino V, Coutris C, Cervoni JP, et al. Prognostic value of C-reactive protein levels in patients with cirrhosis. Liver Transpl. 2015;21(6):753-760.

[119] Michie HR, Manogue KR, Spriggs DR, Roux-Lombard P, J5 Study Group, Lambert PH. Detection of circulating tumor necrosis factor after endotoxin administration. N Engl J Med 1988; 318:1481-1486.

[120] Lisman T, Leebeek FWG, de Groot PG. Haemostatic abnormalitics in patients with liver disease. J Hepatol. 2002;37(2):280-87

[121] Vukovich T, Teufelsbauer H, Fritzer M, Kreuzer S, Knoflach P. Hemostasis activation in patients with liver cirrhosis. Thromb Res. 1995 Feb 1;77(3):271-8.

[122] Tang Z. Zhou JG., Huang WF., Yang MQ. Detection of platelet ca2+ (i), CD62P, CD63 and plasma CD62 P in cirrhosis patients. Chin. J. Hepatol., 2003, 11: 412-414

[123] Violi F, Leo R, Vezza E, Basili S, Cordova C, Balsano F. Bleeding time in patients with cirrhosis-relation with degree of liver failure and clotting abnormalities. C.A.L.C. Group. Coagulation Abnormalities in Cirrhosis Study Group. J. Hepatol., 1994, 20: 531-536

[124] Caldwell SH, Hoffman M, Lisman T, et al. Coagulation disorders and hemostasis in liver disease: pathophysiology and critical assessment of current management. Hepatology. 2006; 44: 1039-1046

[125] Violi F, Basili S, Raparelli V, Chowdary P, Gatt A, Burroughs AK. Patients with liver cirrhosis suffer from primary haemostatic defects? Fact or fiction?. J Hepatol. 2011;55(6):1415-1427.

[126] Monroe DM, Hoffman M. The coagulation cascade in cirrhosis. Clin Liver Dis 2009; 13: 1-9.

[127] Goulis J, Chau TN, Jordan S, Mehta AB, Watkinson A, Rolles K, Burroughs AK. Thrombopoietin concentrations are low in patients with cirrhosis and thrombocytopenia are restored after orthotopic liver transplantation. Gut 1999; 44: 754-8.

[128] Kajihara M, Okazaki Y, Kato S, Ishii H, Kawakami Y, Ikeda Y, Kuwana M. Evaluation of platelet kinetics in patients with liver cirrhosis: similarity to idiopathic thrombocytopenic purpura. J Gastroenterol Hepatol 2007; 22: 112.

[129] Hugenholtz GG, Porte RJ, Lisman T. The platelet and platelet function testing in liver. Disease Clin Liver Dis 2009; 13: 11-20

[130] Thomas DP, Ream VJ, Stuart RK. Platelet aggregation in patients with Laennec's cirrhosis of the liver. N Engl J Med. 1967;276:1344-1348.

[131] Witters P, Freson K, Verslype C, Peerlinck K, Hoylaerts M, Nevens F, et al., Review article: blood platelet number and function in chronic liver disease and cirrhosis. Aliment Pharmacol Ther. 2008;27:1017-1029

[132] Muciño-Bermejo J, Carrillo-Esper R, UribeM,Méndez-SánchezN.Coagulation abnormalities in the cirrhotic patient. Ann Hepatol. 2013;12(5):713-724.

[133] Tripodi A. Hemostasis abnormalities in chronic liver failure. In: Gines P, Kamath PS, Arroyo V, eds. Chronic liver failure: mechanisms and management. New York: Springer, 2010:289-303

[134] Hollestelle MJ, Thinnes T, Crain K, Stiko A, Kruijt JK, van Berkel TJ, et al. Tissue distribution of factor VIII gene expression in vivo – a closer look. Thromb Haemost 2001;86:855-861.

[135] Wion K, Kelly D, Summerfield JA, Tuddenham EG, Lawn RM. Distribution of factor VIII mRNA and antigen in human liver and other tissues. Nature 1985; 317: 726-9.

[136] Shovlin CL, Angus G, Manning RA, Okoli GN, Govani FS, El- derfield K, Birdsey GM, et al. Endothelial cell processing and alternatively spliced transcripts of factor VIII: poten- tial implications for coagulation cascades and pulmonary hypertension. PLoS ONE 2010; 5: 9154.

[137] Wagner DD. Cell biology of von Willebrand factor. Annu Rev Cell Biol 1990; 6: 217-46.

[138] Al Ghumlas AK, Abdel Gader AG, Al Faleh FZ. Haemostatic abnormalities in liver disease: could some haemostatic tests be useful as liver function tests? Blood Coagulation and Fibrinolysis. 2005;16:329-35.

[139] de Maat MP, Nieuwenhuizen W, Knot EA, van Buuren HR, Swart GR. Measuring plasma fibrinogen levels in patients with liver cirrhosis. The occurrence of proteolytic fibrin(ogen) degradation products and their influence on several fibrinogen assays. Thromb Res. 1995 May 15;78(4):353-62. doi: 10.1016/0049-3848(95)91463-u. PMID: 7631315

[140] Amitrano L, Guardascione MA, Brancac-cio V, Balzano A. Coagulation disorders in liver disease. Semin Liver Dis. 2002;22(1):83-96.

[141] Ng VL. Liver disease, coagulation testing, and hemostasis. Clin Lab Med 2009; 29: 265-82.

[142] Dahlback B. Progress in the understanding of the protein C anticoagulant pathway. Int J Hematol 2004;79:109-116

[143] Francis RB Jr, Feinstein DI.Clinical significance of accelerated fibrinolysis in liver disease.Haemostasis. 1984; 14(6): 460-465.

[144] Violi F, Ferro D, Basili S, Quintarelli C, Musca A, Cordova C Balsano F, et al. Hyperfibrinolysis resulting from clotting activation in patients with different degrees of cirrhosis. Hepatology 1993;17:78-83.

[145] Ben Ari Z, Osman E, Hutton RA, Burroughs AK. Disseminated intravascular coagulation in liver cirrhosis: fact or fiction? Am J Gastroenterol 1999;94:2977-2982

[146] Hu KQ, Yu AS, Tiyyagura L, Redeker AG, Reynolds TB. Hyperfibrinolytic activity in hospitalized cirrhotic patients in a referral liver unit. Am J Gastroenterol. 2001 ; 96(5): 1581-1586

[147] Cioni G, Cristani A, Vignoli A, Ventura E. High D-dimer levels: a possible index of risk of overt disseminated intravascular coagulation and/or digestive bleeding in advanced liver cirrhosis?. Recenti Prog Med. 1994;85(4):230-234.

[148] Nilsson T, Wallen P, Mellbring G. In vivo metabolism of human tissue type ptasminogen activator. Scand J Haematol 1984;33: 49-53.

[149] Knot EAR, Drilfhout HR, ten Cate JW, De Jong E, Iburg AHC, Kahle LH, Grijm R. ~2-plasmin inhibitor mechanism in patients with liver cirrhosis. J Lab Clin Med 1985;105:353-358.

[150] Leebeek FWG, Kluft C, Knot EAR, de Maat MPM, Wilson SPH. A shift in balance between profibrinolytic and antifibrinolytic factors causes enhanced fibrinolysis in cirrhosis. Gastroenterology 1991; 101:1382-1390.

[151] Rai V, Dhameja N, Kumar S, Shukla J, Singh R, Dixit VK. Haemostatic Profile of Patients with Chronic Liver Disease- its Correlation with Severity and Outcome. J Clin Diagn Res. 2017;11(8)

[152] Mammen EF. Coagulation abnormalities in liver disease. Haematol Oncol Clin North Am. 1992;6:1247-57.

[153] Deng MH, Liu B, Fang HP, et al. Predictive value of D-dimer for portal vein thrombosis after portal hypertension surgery in hepatitis B virus-related cirrhosis. World J Gastroenterol. 2007;13(48):6588-6592.

[154] Zhang D, Hao J, Yang N. Protein C and D- dimer are related to portal vein thrombosis in pa- tients with liver cirrhosis. J Gastroenterol Hepatol 2010; 25: 116-21.

[155] Dai J, Qi X, Li H, Guo X. Role of D-dimer in the Development of Portal Vein Thrombosis in Liver Cirrhosis: A Meta-analysis. Saudi J Gastroenterol. 2015;21(3):165-174.

[156] Dai J, Qi X, Peng Y, Hou Y, Chen J, Li H, Guo X. Association between D-dimer level and portal venous system thrombosis in liver cirrhosis: a retrospective observational study. Int J Clin Exp Med. 2015 Sep 15;8(9):15296-301. PMID: 26629017; PMCID: PMC4658906.

[157] Primignani M, Dell'Era A, Bucciarelli P, Bottasso B, Bajetta MT, de Franchis R, Cattaneo M. High-D-dimer plasma levels predict poor out-come in esophageal variceal bleeding. Dig Liver Dis 2008; 40: 874-81.

[158] Li Y, Qi X, Li H, Dai J, Deng H, Li J, Peng Y, Liu X, Sun X, Guo X. D-dimer level for predicting the in-hospital mortality in liver cirrhosis: A retrospective study. Exp Ther Med. 2017 Jan;13(1):285-289. doi: 10.3892/etm.2016.3930. Epub 2016 Nov 28. PMID: 28123503; PMCID: PMC5245161.

[159] Violi F, Ferro D, Basili S, et al. Association between low-grade disseminated intravascular coagulation and endotoxemia in patients with liver cirrhosis. Gastroenterology. 1995;109(2):531-539.

[160] Van Deventer SJH, Butler HR, ten Cate JW, Aarden LA, Hack CE, Sturk A. Experimental endotoxemia in humans: analysis of cytokine release and coagulation, fibrinolytic, and complement pathways. Blood 1990;12:2520-2526.

[161] Federici AB, Berkowitz SD, Zimmerman TS, Mannucci PM. Proteolysis of von Willebrand factor after thrombolytic therapy in patients with acute myocardial infarction. Blood 1992;79:38-44.

[162] Atichartarn V, Marder V, Kirby EP, Budzynski AZ. Effects of enzymatic degradation on the subunit composition and biologic properties of human factor VIII. Blood 1978;51:281-292

[163] Semeraro N, Biondi A, Lorenzet R, Locati D, Mantovani A, Donati MB. Direct induction of tissue factor synthesis by endotoxin in human macrophages from diverse anatomical sites. Immunology 1983;50:529-535.

[164] Colucci M, Balconi G, Lorenzet R, Pietra A, Locati D. Cultured human endothelial cells generate tissue factor in response to endotoxins. J Ciin Invest 1983; 71:1893-1896.

[165] Van der Poll T, Buller HR, ten Cate H, Wortel CH, Bauer KA, Van Deventer SJH, Hack E, Sauerwein HP, Rosemberg RD, ten Cate JW. Activation of coagulation after administration of tumor necrosis factor to normal subjects. N Engl J Med 1990;322:1622-1627

[166] Yamamoto K, Shimokawa T, Kojima T, Loskutoff DJ, Saito H. Regulation of murine protein C gene expression in vivo: effects of tumor necrosis factor- alpha, interleukin-1, and transforming growth factor-beta. Thromb Haemost 1999;82:1297-1301.

[167] Palyu E, Harsfalvi J, Tornai T, et al. Major Changes of von Willebrand Factor Multimer Distribution in Cirrhotic Patients with Stable Disease or Acute Decompensation. Thromb Haemost. 2018;118(8):1397-1408

Section 3

Non-Invasive Assessment and Endoscopy in Portal Hypertension

Chapter 5

Non-Invasive Prediction of Gastroesophageal Varices in Patients with Portal Hypertension

Ran Wang, Xiaozhong Guo and Xingshun Qi

Abstract

Gastroesophageal varices are the most common complication of portal hypertension and associated with a worse prognosis. Endoscopy is the gold standard method to diagnose gastroesophageal varices. However, endoscopy is an invasive method with potential complications and is not well adhered by patients. Non-invasive methods, including serum markers or scores, computed tomography, ultrasonographic, and elastography-based methods, have been explored for the diagnosis of gastroesophageal varices. In the current chapter, we will briefly review non-invasive methods for the prediction of gastroesophageal varices.

Keywords: portal hypertension, gastroesophageal varices, non-invasive, diagnosis, prediction

1. Introduction

Portal hypertension is defined as the pressure of portal vein is 5 mmHg higher than that of inferior vena cava. It is the most important complication of liver cirrhosis. Clinically significant portal hypertension is associated with an increased risk of developing varices, which is defined as hepatic venous pressure gradient over 10 mmHg [1]. Gastroesophageal varices (GEVs) is appeared in approximately 50% of patients with cirrhosis, which is associated with a worse outcome. Despite an improvement of treatment strategy, variceal bleeding is still associated with a 6-week mortality rate of 12–26% [2, 3].

Endoscopy, the gold standard method to diagnose GEVs, is recommended for all patients at the time of diagnosis of cirrhosis. Endoscopy should be periodic for screening GEVs. It is reported that nearly 30% of cirrhotic patients screened by endoscopy found to have moderate-to-large varices [4, 5]. Endoscopy is not only a diagnostic method but also serves as a therapeutic option in the form of sclerotherapy and band ligation. However, endoscopy is an invasive method, which is not well perceived by patients. Complications following diagnostic endoscopy mainly include infection, bleeding, duodenal hematoma, bowel perforation, airway obstruction, arrhythmias, and aspiration. Additionally, in some less developed regions or countries, advanced endoscopy and experienced endoscopists are still in shortage. It is thus important to identify patients who can avoid unnecessary endoscopy or patients with high-risk GEVs that need further treatment should be considered.

Non-invasive prediction of GEVs could relieve medical, social, and economic costs. Numerous efforts have been made to predict GEVs non-invasively, and some progress has been achieved. In the Baveno VI consensus conference, it was underlined that non-invasive methods should be used to rule out patients with varices or high-risk varices [6]. In this chapter, we focus on non-invasive methods in the prediction of GEVs.

2. Serum markers or scores

2.1 Serum ammonia

Serum ammonia is well recognized as a serum marker for hepatic encephalopathy in cirrhotic patients. Studies have demonstrated serum ammonia has a positive correlation with the presence of portosystemic collateral veins including GEVs [7]. In a newly published study by **Darweesh et al.** serum ammonia was found significantly higher in patients with esophageal varices (EVs) than those without [8]. A total of 204 hepatitis C virus (HCV) relate cirrhotic patients were enrolled. Serum ammonia with a cutoff value of 82 μmol/L had a sensitivity of 92.3% and specificity of 92% in detecting EVs and that with a cutoff value of 95.5 μmol/L had a sensitivity of 92.7% and specificity of 92.3% in detecting large EVs. Conversely, a study by **Hafez et al.** found that serum ammonia alone cannot predict the presence or grade of EVs [9]. The predictive value of serum ammonia for GEVs still needs further evaluation.

2.2 Platelet count/spleen diameter ratio

Platelet count/spleen diameter ratio (PSR) was first proposed by **Giannini et al.** [10] to explore the non-invasive method for predicting GEVs. In the first part of Giannini's study, 145 patients were included. The results found that PSR was the only parameter independently associated with the EVs with a cutoff value of 909. The PSR with cutoff value of 909 had a sensitivity of 100%, a specificity of 93%, a positive predictive value (PPV) of 96%, and an negative predictive value (NPV) of 100%. In the second part of this study, 103 patients were included, the results validated that the reproducibility of the predictive value of PSR for EVs. Additionally, in all 266 patients, PSR was the only parameter significantly different between patients with and without EVs at baseline.

Since then, extensive studies have focused on the PSR for the non-invasive prediction of GEVs. However, a study by **Schwarzenberger et al.** found PSR maybe not sufficient for the diagnosis of GEVs [11]. In this study, a total of 137 patients were enrolled. The diameter of spleen was measured using computed tomography (CT), magnetic resonance imaging, and ultrasonography. Ascites, splenomegaly, Child-Pugh score were found to have a positive correlation with EVs. The PSR with a cutoff of 909 had a sensitivity of 80%, specificity of 66%, and PPV of 74%.

In a recent meta-analysis by **Chen et al.** where 49 studies were enrolled, found that the area under curves (AUC) of PSR for GEVs was 0.8719, the summary sensitivity and specificity were 0.84 and 0.78, respectively [12]. The results suggest that PSR can be used for predicting EVs, especially in patients with viral hepatitis.

2.3 Liaoning score

The Liaoning score was proposed by **Qi et al.** from a prospective cohort of cirrhotic patients who underwent the first-time endoscopy at 11 hospitals in Liaoning

Province, China [13]. In this study, a total of 363 cirrhotic patients were enrolled. The incidence of EVs was 71.63% (260/363). The results suggest that acute upper gastrointestinal bleeding (AUGIB), platelet count, and ascites were independently associated with the presence of EVs. In the whole cirrhotic patients, the Liaoning score, whose equation was $0.466 + 1.088 \times$ AUGIB (1 = yes; 0 = no) $+ 1.147 \times$ ascites (1 = yes; 0 = no) $- 0.012 \times$ platelet count, had an AUC of 0.807 ($p < 0.0001$). The cutoff value was 0.474 with a sensitivity of 70%, a specificity of 77.67%, a PPV of 88.8%, and an NPV of 50.6%. In patients with AUGIB, the equation was $1.205 + 1.557 \times$ ascites (1 = yes; 0 = no) $- 0.008 \times$ platelet count, with an AUC of 0.782 ($p < 0.0001$). The results of this study suggested that Liaoning score was a newly developed scoring system which can be employed to predict EVs in cirrhotic patients.

For external validation of Liaoning score, **Li et al.** performed a nationwide multicenter cross-sectional study to evaluate the predictive ability of Liaoning score for EVs and high-risk EVs [14]. In this study, 612 cirrhotic patients with AUGIB were enrolled. The incidence of EVs and high-risk EVs was 96.2% and 95.6%, respectively. The results showed that the AUC of Liaoning score for predicting EVs was 0.708 ($p = 0.0016$), and that of high-risk EVs was 0.702 ($p = 0.0147$).

2.4 Other scores

Other than the non-invasive methods we have discussed above, many scores have been developed for the evaluation of liver fibrosis, including aspartate aminotransferase-to-platelet ratio index (APRI), aspartate aminotransferase-to-alanine aminotransferase ratio (AAR), FIB-4, and Lok scores. Some studies explore the predictive ability of these non-invasive scores for GEVs. In a meta-analysis by **Deng et al.** several non-invasive scores had been systematically reviewed for the predictive ability of EVs [15]. In the overall analysis, a total of 650 patients were included, 81.4% of them had moderate–severe EVs. Only Child-Pugh and FI scores were significantly higher in patients with EVs than those without. The AUC of FI was 0.612, FIB-4 was 0.567, AAR was 0.56, and APRI was 0.539. However, the AUC among these scores was not significantly different. For further validation, **Deng et al.** also performed a retrospective study, the results were in agreement with their previous meta-analysis [16]. A total of 650 cirrhotic patients were included, and 81.4% of them had high-risk EVs. The results of this study concluded that APRI, AAR, and FIB-4 scores had only modest diagnostic accuracy of EVs in cirrhotic patients.

3. Image tools

3.1 CT

CT scanning is one of the most important image tools in clinical practice, is recommended for the surveillance of hepatocellular carcinoma in all cirrhotic patients. GEVs characteristics as round, tubular, or serpentine structures in the esophagus and/or gastric lumen in CT images. It provides a possibility that an experienced physician can diagnosis GEVs using CT images, especially in contrast-enhanced CT images.

Perri et al. designed a prospective study that explores the ability of CT for the prediction of GEVs [5]. A total of 102 patients who had a CT and endoscopy within 5 days were enrolled. Two radiologists read the CT independently. The sensitivity of EVs was 93% in both radiologists, the specificity was 55% and 45%, respectively. The sensitivity of gastric varices was 87% in both radiologists. The results suggest that CT should be used as initial surveillance for GEVs.

In a study by **Li et al.** contrast-enhanced CT was used for the non-invasive prediction of GEVs [17]. In this retrospectively study, a total of 279 patients were included. High-risk varices including EVs and gastric varices was defined as varices that need treatment. All patients were divided into four groups according to the history of bleeding events, endoscopic surveillance, and drug prophylaxis (primary or secondary prophylaxis). In the overall population, only contrast-enhanced CT was significantly associated with EVs, high-risk EVs, and gastric varices. In primary prophylaxis, acute bleeding, previous bleeding, and secondary prophylaxis population, a diameter < 0.5 cm, <0.38 cm <0.46 cm and < 0.33 cm was considered as the cut-off value of high-risk EVs, respectively. Which can spare 47.8%, 10.5%, 12.1%, and 7.8% of endoscopic surveillance with no high-risk EVs was missed, respectively. This study showed a good diagnostic performance for contrast-enhanced CT for patients with GEVs.

3.2 Ultrasonography

Ultrasonography is the most common, cost-effective, and convenient imaging tool in clinical practice, which can be used for screening of hepatocellular carcinoma, measure the width of the portal vein, inferior vena cava, and diameter of the spleen.

Splenoportal index was calculated as the splenic index divided by mean portal vein velocity. In a study by **Mansoor et al.** 200 HCV-induced cirrhotic patients were included [18]. All patients underwent ultrasonography first to calculate splenoportal index and then underwent endoscopy. The incidence of EVs was 60.5% (121/200) in ultrasonography and 63.5% (127/200) in endoscopy. The sensitivity, specificity, PPV, NPV of ultrasonography for predicting EVs was 88.98%, 89.04%, 93.00%, 82.28%, and 89.00%, respectively. This study showed a good diagnostic performance for splenoportal index by ultrasonography for patients with EVs.

3.3 Elastography-based methods

Elastography-based methods, Including transient elastography (TE), point shear wave elastography, two-dimensional shear wave elastography, and magnetic resonance elastography have been used to non-invasively detected liver fibrosis and GEVs. There is substantial evidence suggesting that TE had a good correlation with portal hypertension and varices in cirrhotic patients [19, 20]. In 2015, TE was recommended for the surveillance of GEVs by Baveno VI consensus [6]. According to the Baveno VI consensus, in patients with compensated advanced chronic liver disease, who had a liver stiffness <20 kPa measured by TE and platelet count >150,000/mm^3, had a low risk of developed GEVs that may spear endoscopy. **Augustin et al.** performed a prospective study that taking the Baveno VI recommendation a step forward [21]. This study suggests that platelet count >110,000/mm^3 and liver stiffness <25 kPa can spare more endoscopies than the Baveno VI consensus recommendation (41% vs. 21%). Only minority (0.6%) of overall patients were missed varices needing treatment. The negative predictive value for varices of the Baveno VI consensus and expanded Baveno VI consensus criteria is confirmed by further studies [22, 23].

In a study by **Kim et al.** a new model was generate based on the liver elasticity and the spleen diameter/platelet count (LSPS) [24]. A total of 280 hepatitis B virus relate cirrhotic patients were enrolled into the training cohort, and 121 patients were enrolled into the validation cohort. Liver stiffness was measured by TE. LSPS was calculated by the equation: Liver Stiffness Measurement × spleen diameter/platelet count. In the training cohort, the cutoff value of LSPS was 3.5. In patients with LSPS <3.5, the absence of high-risk EVs had a sensitivity of 87.7%, a specificity of 91.1%, an NPV of 94%, and a PPV of 82.3%. When applying the cutoff value of LSPS <3.5, the AUC in the validation cohorts was 0.953. The results of this study showed that in patients with LSPS <3.5, endoscopy may avoid safely in cirrhotic patients.

In a study by **Sharma et al.** spleen stiffness was used for the non-invasive prediction of GEVs [25]. A total of 174 cirrhotic patients were prospectively enrolled. Liver stiffness and spleen stiffness were measured by the TE. Median liver stiffness, median spleen stiffness, LSPS, and PSR were significantly different between patients with and without EVs. On multivariate analysis, only liver stiffness and spleen stiffness showed predictive ability of EVs. Liver stiffness with a cutoff value of 27.3 kPa had a higher AUC than spleen stiffness with a cutoff value of 40.8 kPa (0.908 vs. 0.898). The liver stiffness with a cutoff value of ≥27.3 kPa had a sensitivity of 91%, a specificity of 72%, a PPV of 89%, an NPV of 76%, and a diagnostic accuracy of 86% in predicting EVs; the spleen stiffness with a cutoff of ≥40.8 kPa had a sensitivity of 94%, a specificity of 76%, a PPV of 91%, an NPV of 84%, and a diagnostic accuracy of 86% in predicting EVs. In patients who had performed hepatic venous pressure gradient, spleen stiffness showed a correlation with hepatic venous pressure gradient ($r = 0.335$, $P = 0.01$). The results of this study suggest that spleen stiffness can be used for the non-invasive assessment of EVs.

4. Discussion

GEVs exists in almost 30–60% of cirrhotic patients, depending on the severity of portal hypertension [24]. The occurrence of GEVs and varices-related AUGIB significantly worsened the prognosis of patients with portal hypertension, emphasizes the importance of diagnosis and management of GEVs. There are numerous studies have focused on developing non-invasive methods to predict the presence of GEVs, including serum markers, CT scanning, and ultrasonographic parameters. However, endoscopy is still difficult to replace, especially considering cost-effectiveness and diagnostic accuracy [26]. From other perspectives, in regular physical examination or surveillance of hepatocellular carcinoma, non-invasive methods can be employed to predict the severity of portal hypertension and GEVs. In this situation, if the patients have a high-risk of variceal bleeding in a short time, then the patient must perform endoscopy; if the patient has a low-risk of bleeding in a certain period, then the patient can waive an unnecessary endoscopy.

Liver stiffness and spleen stiffness measured by the TE were the most promising non-invasive methods available, as they have proven having a good correlation with liver fibrosis, portal hypertension, and the presence with varices [27, 28]. The limitations of TE is that the results of TE should interpreted by a specialist in liver disease which may not available in less development hospital and TE should inappropriate be performed in patients with ascites and/or obesity [26].

Approximately 10% of the whole portal hypertension patients were non-cirrhotic portal hypertension [29]. In general, patients with non-cirrhotic portal hypertension have higher prevalence and larger size of varices than those in cirrhotic patients [30, 31]. Until now, few studies focus on the non-invasive prediction of GEVs in patients with non-cirrhotic portal hypertension. In a retrospective observational study by **Cunningham et al.** [32] a total of 44 non-cirrhotic portal hypertension patients were enrolled, and 15 of them had high-risk varices. The results of this study found that spleen diameter > 17.2 cm had a sensitivity of 78.6% and specificity of 64.3% for prediction of high-risk varices. In patients with non-cirrhotic portal hypertension, the LSM and PSR may not as useful as cirrhotic patients.

There are heterogeneities among these studies and methods. Several reasons for the heterogeneities, including: 1) different target populations were enrolled among studies, including different races, etiology of liver cirrhosis; 2) different severity of underlying liver disease among patients; 3) different definitions for the risk of GEVs: in some studies, such as the study by **Li et al**. the severity of EVs was defined using the shape of varices and the red color sign [17]; in some other studies, the severity of varices was defined using the size of varices [5]. Therefore, the heterogeneities make it difficult to compare different studies or methods systematically.

5. Conclusion

Endoscopy is still the first choice for the diagnosis of GEVs in patients with portal hypertension. Liver stiffness and spleen stiffness measured by TE are the most studied methods. With the development of non-invasive prediction of GEVs, it is promising to exempt some patients from endoscopy.

Author details

Ran Wang*, Xiaozhong Guo and Xingshun Qi
Department of Gastroenterology, General Hospital of Northern Theater Command, Shenyang, China

*Address all correspondence to: wangran891017@163.com

References

[1] Garcia-Tsao, G., et al., *Portal hypertensive bleeding in cirrhosis: Risk stratification, diagnosis, and management: 2016 practice guidance by the American Association for the study of liver diseases.* Hepatology, 2017. **65**(1): p. 310-335.

[2] Fortune, B.E., et al., *Child-Turcotte-Pugh Class is Best at Stratifying Risk in Variceal Hemorrhage: Analysis of a US Multicenter Prospective Study.* J Clin Gastroenterol, 2017. **51**(5): p. 446-453.

[3] Lee, H.H., et al., *A simplified prognostic model to predict mortality in patients with acute variceal bleeding.* Dig Liver Dis, 2018. **50**(3): p. 247-253.

[4] Zaman, A., et al., *Prevalence of upper and lower gastrointestinal tract findings in liver transplant candidates undergoing screening endoscopic evaluation.* Am J Gastroenterol, 1999. **94**(4): p. 895-899.

[5] Perri, R.E., et al., *A prospective evaluation of computerized tomographic (CT) scanning as a screening modality for esophageal varices.* Hepatology, 2008. **47**(5): p. 1587-1594.

[6] de Franchis, R. and V.I.F. Baveno, *Expanding consensus in portal hypertension: Report of the Baveno VI Consensus Workshop: Stratifying risk and individualizing care for portal hypertension.* J Hepatol, 2015. **63**(3): p. 743-752.

[7] Tarantino, G., et al., *Blood ammonia levels in liver cirrhosis: a clue for the presence of portosystemic collateral veins.* BMC Gastroenterol, 2009. **9**: p. 21.

[8] Darweesh, S.K., et al., *Serum ammonia as a non-invasive marker for early prediction of esophageal varices.* Eur J Gastroenterol Hepatol, 2021. **32**(2): p. 230-236.

[9] Hafez, H.A., *Predictive value of non-invasive blood ammonia level for the presence of oesophageal varices in Egyptian patients with liver cirrhosis.* Journal of Gastroenterology, 2015. **4**(5): p. 1613-1617.

[10] Giannini, E., et al., *Platelet count/spleen diameter ratio: proposal and validation of a non-invasive parameter to predict the presence of oesophageal varices in patients with liver cirrhosis.* Gut, 2003. **52**(8): p. 1200-1205.

[11] Schwarzenberger, E., et al., *Utilization of platelet count spleen diameter ratio in predicting the presence of esophageal varices in patients with cirrhosis.* J Clin Gastroenterol, 2010. **44**(2): p. 146-150.

[12] Chen, R., et al., *Platelet Count to Spleen Diameter Ratio for the Diagnosis of Gastroesophageal Varices in Liver Cirrhosis: A Systematic Review and Meta-Analysis.* Gastroenterol Res Pract, 2017. **2017**: p. 7407506.

[13] Qi, X., et al., *Liaoning Score for Prediction of Esophageal Varices in Cirrhotic Patients Who Had Never Undergone Endoscopy: A Multicenter Cross-Sectional Study in Liaoning Province, China.* Adv Ther, 2019. **36**(8): p. 2167-2178.

[14] Li, Q., et al., *External validation of Liaoning score for predicting esophageal varices in liver cirrhosis: a Chinese multicenter cross-sectional study.* Ann Transl Med, 2019. **7**(23): p. 755.

[15] Deng, H., X. Qi, and X. Guo, *Diagnostic Accuracy of APRI, AAR, FIB-4, FI, King, Lok, Forns, and FibroIndex Scores in Predicting the Presence of Esophageal Varices in Liver Cirrhosis: A Systematic Review and Meta-Analysis.* Medicine (Baltimore), 2015. **94**(42): p. e1795.

[16] Deng, H., et al., *Diagnostic Accuracy of APRI, AAR, FIB-4, FI, and King Scores*

for Diagnosis of Esophageal Varices in Liver Cirrhosis: A Retrospective Study. Med Sci Monit, 2015. **21**: p. 3961-3977.

[17] Li, Q., et al., *Contrast-Enhanced CT May Be a Diagnostic Alternative for Gastroesophageal Varices in Cirrhosis with and without Previous Endoscopic Variceal Therapy.* Gastroenterol Res Pract, 2019. **2019**: p. 6704673.

[18] Mansoor, A., et al., *Diagnostic Accuracy of Doppler Ultrasonography in Predicting Presence of Esophageal Varices in Patients with Hepatitis-C Induced Cirrhosis.* J Coll Physicians Surg Pak, 2019. **29**(7): p. 612-615.

[19] Jangouk, P., et al., *Validating, deconstructing and refining Baveno criteria for ruling out high-risk varices in patients with compensated cirrhosis.* Liver Int, 2017. **37**(8): p. 1177-1183.

[20] Maurice, J.B., et al., *Validation of the Baveno VI criteria to identify low risk cirrhotic patients not requiring endoscopic surveillance for varices.* J Hepatol, 2016. **65**(5): p. 899-905.

[21] Augustin, S., et al., *Expanding the Baveno VI criteria for the screening of varices in patients with compensated advanced chronic liver disease.* Hepatology, 2017. **66**(6): p. 1980-1988.

[22] Giannini, E.G., et al., *Course of oesophageal varices and performance of noninvasive predictors following Hepatitis C Virus clearance in compensated advanced chronic liver disease.* Eur J Clin Invest, 2020. **50**(5): p. e13231.

[23] Gaete, M.I., et al., *Baveno VI and Expanded Baveno VI criteria successfully predicts the absence of high-risk gastro-oesophageal varices in a Chilean cohort.* Liver Int, 2020. **40**(6): p. 1427-1434.

[24] Kim, B.K., et al., *A liver stiffness measurement-based, noninvasive prediction model for high-risk esophageal varices in B-viral liver cirrhosis.* Am J Gastroenterol, 2010. **105**(6): p. 1382-1390.

[25] Sharma, P., et al., *Spleen stiffness in patients with cirrhosis in predicting esophageal varices.* Am J Gastroenterol, 2013. **108**(7): p. 1101-7.

[26] European Association for Study of, L. and H. Asociacion Latinoamericana para el Estudio del, *EASL-ALEH Clinical Practice Guidelines: Non-invasive tests for evaluation of liver disease severity and prognosis.* J Hepatol, 2015. **63**(1): p. 237-264.

[27] Carrion, J.A., et al., *Transient elastography for diagnosis of advanced fibrosis and portal hypertension in patients with hepatitis C recurrence after liver transplantation.* Liver Transpl, 2006. **12**(12): p. 1791-1798.

[28] Lemoine, M., et al., *Liver stiffness measurement as a predictive tool of clinically significant portal hypertension in patients with compensated hepatitis C virus or alcohol-related cirrhosis.* Aliment Pharmacol Ther, 2008. **28**(9): p. 1102-1110.

[29] Simonetto, D.A., M. Liu, and P.S. Kamath, *Portal Hypertension and Related Complications: Diagnosis and Management.* Mayo Clin Proc, 2019. **94**(4): p. 714-726.

[30] Madhu, K., et al., *Idiopathic non-cirrhotic intrahepatic portal hypertension: common cause of cryptogenic intrahepatic portal hypertension in a Southern Indian tertiary hospital.* Indian J Gastroenterol, 2009. **28**(3): p. 83-87.

[31] Dhiman, R.K., et al., *Non-cirrhotic portal fibrosis (idiopathic portal hypertension): experience with 151 patients and a review of the literature.* J Gastroenterol Hepatol, 2002. **17**(1): p. 6-16.

[32] Cunningham, M.E., et al., *Noninvasive Predictors of High-Risk Varices in Patients with Non-Cirrhotic Portal Hypertension.* Can J Gastroenterol Hepatol, 2019. **2019**: p. 1808797.

Chapter 6

Endoscopy in Management of Portal Hypertension

Bhavik Bharat Shah, Usha Goenka and Mahesh Kumar Goenka

Abstract

Portal hypertension (PH) is a serious consequence of several disease states affecting prehepatic, intrahepatic, or posthepatic portal circulation. Backpressure caused by PH transmits through the collaterals to form varices at various sites. PH also leads to hyperdynamic congestion and altered gastrointestinal mucosal immune response, resulting in portal hypertensive gastropathy (PHG), portal hypertensive enteropathy (PHE), and portal colopathy (PC). These PH associated phenomena may lead to torrential life-threatening bleed or chronic blood loss leading to debilitating chronic anemia. Endoscopy plays a pivotal role in the management of these patients both for diagnostic and therapeutic purpose. The choice of therapeutic strategy depends on many factors: severity of the disease, patient's clinical performance, and whether it is done as an emergency or as a prophylactic approach. In this chapter, we evaluate the endoscopic management of patients with the gastrointestinal complications of PH.

Keywords: portal hypertension, esophageal varices, gastric varices, portal hypertensive gastropathy, gastric antral vascular ectasia, portal hypertensive enteropathy, portal colopathy

1. Introduction

Portal hypertension (PH) is a serious consequence of disease states affecting prehepatic, intrahepatic, or posthepatic portal circulation. Liver cirrhosis, which leads to sinusoidal hypertension, is the most frequent etiology of PH. Cirrhosis causes structural distortion in the liver architecture accompanied by the rise in local intrahepatic vasoconstrictors. Cirrhosis also causes an increase in systemic vasodilation and increased cardiac output leading to increased portal blood flow. When portal pressure, measured as hepatic vein portal gradient (HPVG), is >10 mm of Hg, it leads to development of portosystemic collaterals (**Figure 1**). These collaterals arise due to recanalization of fetal vascular channels, reversal of flow within adult veins, and/or because of neoangiogenesis [1]. Backpressure caused by PH transmits through these collaterals to perforating veins and the submucosal vessels they supply, whereby varices may form.

A PH related increase in the portal vein pressure leads to hyperdynamic congestion in the gastric, small intestinal, and colonic mucosa. The mucosa undergoes microcirculatory changes, such as submucosal angiogenesis and vascular ectasia, that impair its integrity and promote its susceptibility to damage. Moreover, local

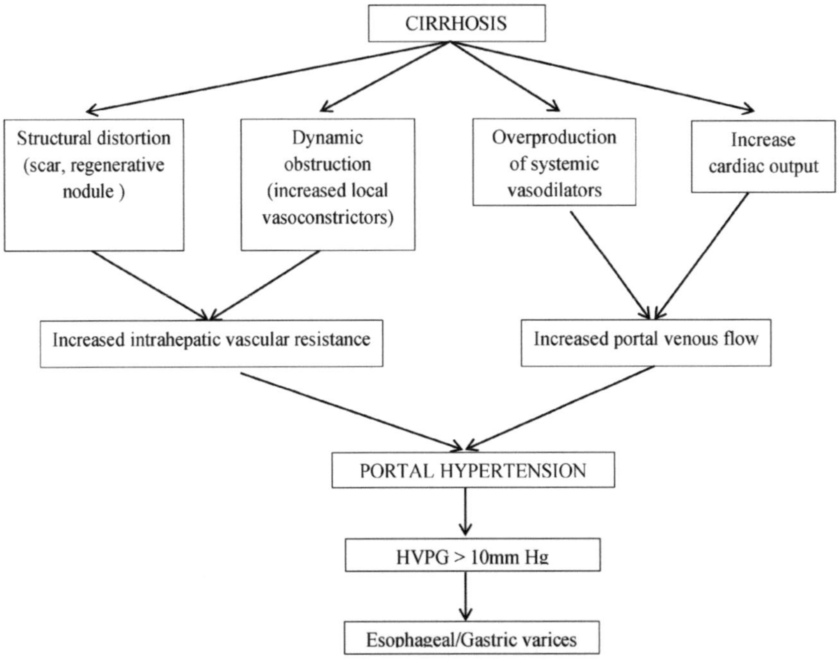

Figure 1.
Pathophysiology of formation of varices in cirrhosis.

immune mucosal defense mechanisms are impaired in PH. All these lead to portal hypertensive gastropathy (PHG), portal hypertensive enteropathy (PHE), and portal colopathy (PC) [2, 3]. This chapter focuses on the endoscopic management of varices, PHG, Gastric antral vascular ectasia (GAVE), PHE, and PC.

2. Esophageal varices

Esophageal varices are present in 30–40% of patients with Child A cirrhosis and approximately 85% of those with Child B/C cirrhosis [4]. Despite improved surveillance and treatment, the rate of variceal hemorrhage (VH) continues to be 10–15% per year, with an 6-week mortality of 15–25% [5]. Mortality risk is particularly high when VH is associated with acute kidney injury (AKI) and/or concomitant bacterial infections [6]. Recurrent VH occurs in 60% of patients without treatment [7].

Considering the high-risk of death when VH occurs, implementing surveillance strategies to prevent bleeding and death should be pursued actively in patients with cirrhosis. Once the patient is diagnosed with cirrhosis, a periodic surveillance endoscopy is warranted to look for esophageal varices. Other modalities such as video capsule endoscopy (VCE), computed tomography (CT) scan, or Fibroscan have been assessed for their role in detecting esophageal varices [8, 9]. However, endoscopy is still regarded as the investigation of choice.

2.1 Primary prophylaxis

The risk factors of VH are the large size of varices, red signs, and the severity of liver disease [10]. Primary prophylaxis must be initiated in "high-risk varices" **(Figure 2a)**. This includes small varices (<5 mm) with red color signs, any varix in Child-C patients or large varices (>5 mm) irrespective of Child-Pugh

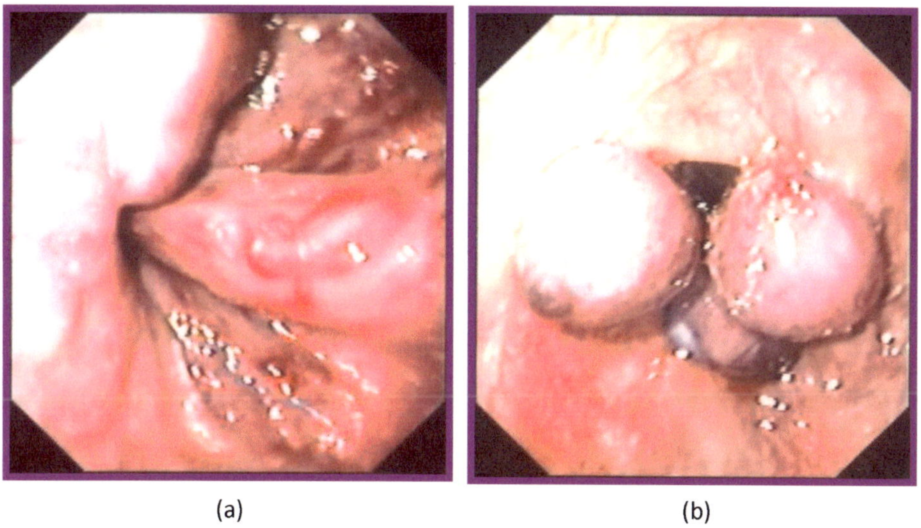

Figure 2.
Endoscopic appearance of esophageal varix. (a) Large esophageal varix with red color signs, (b) esophageal varix after endoscopic band ligation.

classification [11]. In patients with "low-risk varices" or no varices, surveillance endoscopy should be undertaken at interval of 2–3 years, depending on the severity of the liver disease and whether the liver injury is ongoing or not (**Figure 3**). The patients with active alcoholism, non-alcoholic steatohepatitis (NASH), hepatitis B and C with detectable viral load are some examples of ongoing liver injury.

The primary prophylaxis of "high-risk varices" involves pharmacological prophylaxis using a nonselective beta-adrenergic blockers (NSBB) or endoscopic band ligation (EVL). NSBBs such as propranolol and nadolol reduce cardiac output and splanchnic blood flow through nonselective beta-blockade, and the unopposed effect of alpha-1 adrenergic receptors leads to splanchnic vasoconstriction. This reduces the portal pressure and its consequential complications. Carvedilol, an NSBB with

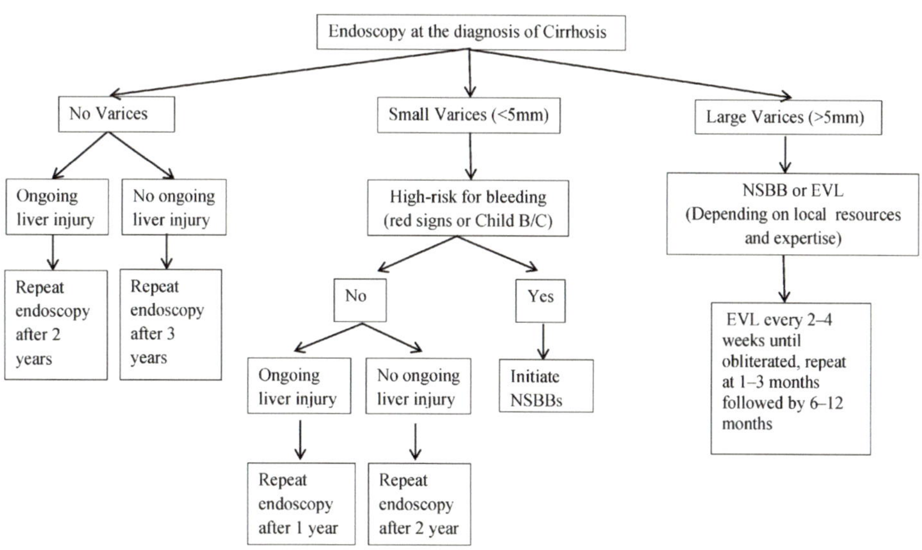

Figure 3.
Algorithm for surveillance and primary prophylaxis of esophageal varix.

intrinsic anti-alpha-1 receptor activity, reduces both porto-collateral and intrahepatic resistance. However, this is at the cost of more profound effects on the systemic arterial pressure, particularly in decompensated patients. Carvedilol is therefore, preferred in patients where NSSB are contraindicated or produce side effect.

EVL (**Figure 2b**) involves the placement of rubber rings on variceal columns, which are sucked into a plastic hollow cylinder attached to the endoscope tip. Ligation causes occlusion of the varix and subsequent thrombosis with ischemic necrosis of the mucosa. Band placement should be limited to the distal 8 cm segment of the esophagus in order to target the palisade drainage and perforating zones. Bands should be placed helically, moving distal to proximal to allow the maximum number of bands to be applied while avoiding overlapping circumferential placement. More proximal placement has less efficacy and may cause post ligation retrosternal discomfort. Complications after EBL occur in approximately 2–20% of the patients and include transient dysphagia, retrosternal pain, esophageal stricture, ulceration, perforation, and infection [12]. Occasionally, massive bleeding can occur, either from recurrent variceal rupture or from post-ligation ulceration.

It is generally recommended that small varices with red signs should be treated with NSBBs. Large varices can be treated with either NSBBs or EBL. The treatment choice is based on local resource and expertise, patient preference, contraindications, and adverse events [11, 13, 14].

2.2 Acute esophageal variceal hemorrhage (AVH)

Ruptured esophageal varices contributes to 70% of all the upper gastrointestinal (GI) bleeding episodes in patients with portal hypertension [15]. Initial treatment should always target restoring the euvolemic status. Restrictive blood transfusion strategy is adequate in most patients with GI bleed [16]. Vasoactive drug therapy and antibiotic prophylaxis should be initiated as soon as AVH is suspected [11]. After adequate resuscitation, an endoscopic evaluation should be carried out in patients with acute variceal bleed, in the first 12 hours after admission [13]. **Table 1** shows various modalities which can be used to treat esophageal variceal bleed.

2.3 Endoscopic variceal band ligation (EVL)

EVL is the preferred endoscopic therapy for active bleeding, as it allows greater bleeding control, with lower adverse events, and improves survival compared to endoscopic sclerotherapy (ES) which was practiced earlier [17]. In AVH, EVL should be preferentially targeted toward the culprit variceal column evidenced by the ongoing ooze or presence of stigmata of hemorrhage. However, during active

Endoscopic Therapy
• Variceal band ligation (EVL)
• Sclero therapy/ Glue injection
• Tamponade using
○ SB tube
○ Metal stents
• Argon plasma coagulation
TIPS

Table 1.
Therapeutic options for control of acute esophageal variceal bleed.

bleeding, banding at the gastroesophageal junction may reduce bleeding, allowing visualization and appropriate targeting of subsequent bands.

Despite adequate therapy with vasoactive drugs combined with EVL, up to 10–15% of patients with variceal hemorrhage have persistent bleeding or early rebleeding [18]. Transjugular intrahepatic portosystemic shunts (TIPS) should be considered as a rescue therapy of choice in this group of patients [13]. When TIPS is not feasible or in case of modest rebleeding, a second endoscopic therapy with repeat EVL or alternate methods may be attempted, and vasoactive drugs doses should also be optimized.

2.4 Endoscopic sclerotherapy and glue injection

The sclerosant injection acts by precipitating inflammation and thrombosis of the varix. ES involves intravariceal injection of sclerosant at and just distal to the site of the bleeding, or perivariceal injection performed adjacent to a varix. Injection should be first performed at the bleeding site, followed by perivariceal or intravariceal injection starting from the GE junction, with proximal injections at 2-cm intervals, extending up to 5 cm to 6 cm from the GE junction. Sclerosants used include sodium tetradecyl sulfate (Food and Drug Administration approved), sodium morrhuate, ethanolamine oleate, polidocanol, or absolute alcohol.

A meta-analysis of 14 studies found that EVL is better than ES in terms of lower rates of rebleeding and complications and a higher rate of variceal eradication [19]. The complications related to ES occur in up to 40% of patients, and include esophageal ulceration, stricture, perforation, pleural effusion, hemothorax, pulmonary thromboembolism, pericarditis, mediastinitis, pneumothorax, renal dysfunction, and even death [20]. Though EVL is the therapy of choice for the management of bleeding varices, there are a few indications where EVL is technically demanding, and ES can be utilized. This includes massive ongoing bleed when visualization is impaired, when adequate tissue suctioning into the cap is not possible due to scar, and in young children.

Glue injection have also been performed for active variceal bleeding. Overall, there is no definitive evidence supporting the use of cyanoacrylate injection for the management of bleeding varices or for VH prophylaxis. Tissue adhesive injection may be considered in conjunction with sclerotherapy. However, a RCT did show that using n-butyl cyanoacrylate and sclerosant injection in conjunction, resulted in lower rebleeding and mortality compared to using sclerotherapy alone [21].

2.5 Tamponade using balloons or metal stents

For persistent VH, where EVL has failed, as well as for EVL-related ulcer bleeding, balloon tamponade (BT) using Sengstaken-Blakemore (SB) tube and emergency TIPS have been advocated [13]. SB tube is associated with many complications and rebound bleeding. Performing TIPS in emergencies may not be feasible in many centres. Besides, there are cost issues and a definite risk of encephalopathy in the presence of advanced liver dysfunction [22]. Covered self-expanding metal stents (SEMS) with distinctive designs are used to produce an effective tamponade, controlling persistent variceal bleeding and ulcer bleeding following VBL [23, 24].

Initially, the Choo stent (diameter 18 mm, length 140 mm, NES – 18 – 080 – 070, MI Tech Co., Ltd) and the EllaBoubella-Danis stent (diameter 20 mm, length 95 mm, Ella-CS, Hradec Kralove, Czech Republic) were used. Despite demonstrating efficacy, these stent designs were not ideal for deployment and use in variceal bleeding; hence the SX-ELLA Danis Stent (Ella-CS, Hradec Kralove, Czech Republic) was designed [23]. SX_ELLA Danis Stent (**Figure 4**) is the most commonly used

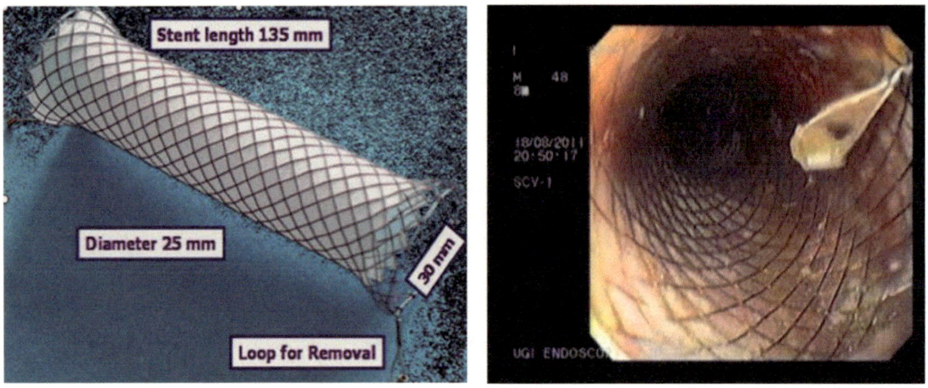

Figure 4.
Ela stent: SX ELLA STENT. A) Stent design, B) stent in esophagus.

stent for the treatment of persistent VH. It differs from the Choo stent and the EllaBoubela-Danis stent in having a balloon-style delivery system. These stents are made of nitinol, measuring 13.5 cm in length with a diameter of 25 mm in the shaft and 30 mm at the ends. The stents are placed usually over an endoscopically placed guidewire but can also be inserted at bedside without the need of an endoscope. The stent's unique delivery system uses a gastric positioning balloon placed just distal to caudal end of the stent. The correct positioning of the stent in the distal half of the esophagus is established by inflating the gastric balloon and retracting the catheter assembly until the gastric balloon hits against the cardia. The stent is then released, and the gastric balloon is deflated, and the assembly catheter is removed [24]. These stents act by causing a steady mechanical compression causing an immediate tamponade at the variceal bleed site. Compared to SB tube, these stents allow oral feeding and endoscopic assessment of rebleed.

In a meta-analysis of 12 studies, which evaluated SEMS placement for refractory esophageal variceal hemorrhage, the reported clinical success (absence of bleeding within 24 hours of SEMS placement) rate was 96% (95% CI, 0.90–1.00) and technical success (guidewire-assisted endoscopic SEMS deployment) rate was 97% (95% CI, 0.91–1.00). Adverse events associated with the placement of SEMS include stent migration (28%), rebleeding (16%), and ulcer. However, there was no significant difference in mortality compared to balloon tamponade [25]. Removal of SX-ELLA Danis stent is advised within 2 weeks following stent insertion, under endoscopic guidance using the custom PEXElla extractor (Ella-CS) or usual foreign body forceps [26].

2.6 Argon plasma coagulation (APC)

APC is an electrosurgery-based, non-contact, multi-directional coagulation method. A high-frequency current is applied to the target tissue through an argon plasma jet with a constant depth of energy penetration (maximum 4 mm). APC has been used to coagulate the distal esophageal mucosa after eradicating esophageal varices by endoscopic variceal ligation to reduce the rate of variceal recurrence and need for rebanding. This technique is generally recommended as secondary prophylaxis for esophageal variceal bleeding in those who have contraindications, are intolerant, or are non-compliant to NSSB [27]. A meta-analysis of four randomized controlled trials (RCT) compared the safety and efficacy of EVL alone, with EVL along with APC, for secondary prophylaxis of esophageal variceal bleeding. Across the 4 RCTs, combination therapy showed significantly lower variceal recurrence rates (relative risk 0.19). There was no difference in re-bleeding or mortality. Fever occurred more often after combination therapy [28].

After ensuring the complete eradication of varices, APC is initiated 2 to 3 weeks after the last EVL session. APC is generally performed at a gas flow rate of 1.2–2 L/min. The power setting of the APC current generator is adjusted at 50 to 70 W. The entire esophageal mucosa proximal to the esophageal junction is coagulated with APC in 2 sessions at 2-week intervals. In each session, one half of the mucosa is ablated thermally starting at the esophagogastric junction by retracting the probe proximally, while delivering thermal energy creating longitudinal parallel stripes of coagulated tissue.

3. Gastric varices

Gastric varices (GV) are the source of bleeding in 5–10% of patients with PH, second only to the esophageal variceal bleed [15]. GV is, however, relatively more common in non-cirrhotic portal hypertension (NCPH) and extrahepatic portal vein obstruction (EHPVO) occurring in 1/4th and 1/3rd of patients, respectively [20].

The GV classification system aligns with the therapeutic distinction and categorizes GV based on whether they are contiguous with esophageal varices or not, and as per their location in the stomach (**Figure 5**) [29]. Gastroesophageal varices (GOV) are contiguous with the esophageal varices extending either into the lesser curvature (GOV1) or the fundus along the greater curvature (GOV2). These varices share the pathophysiology of esophageal varices, arising from the left gastric vein and originate in the lamina propria. Isolated Gastric Varices (IGV) are distinct from GOV and can be located either in the cardia (IGV1) or outside of the cardia and fundus, usually the antrum or pylorus (IGV2). These arise from the short and posterior gastric veins and originate in the submucosa.

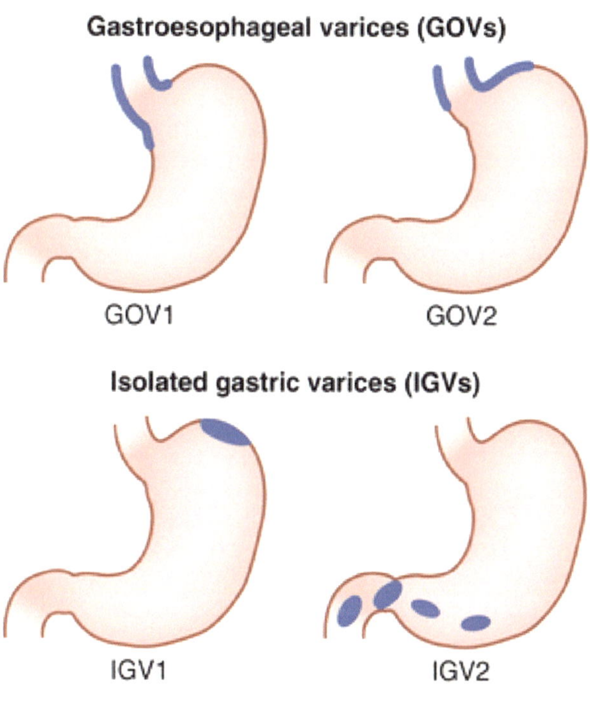

Figure 5.
Sarin Classifiaction of gastric varix. GOV- gastroesophageal varix, IGV- isolated gastric varix.

Gastric variceal bleeding (**Figure 6**), although less common, has the predisposition to be more severe, associated with higher blood transfusion requirement, and increased morbidity, and mortality compared with esophageal variceal bleeding [30]. The probable cause for this is a large submucosal component of GV, the vascular structures feeding and draining the gastric varix, and, also, the lack of widespread expertise. Bleeding risk is significantly higher for the IGV1 (77%) and GOV2 (55%), than for GOV1 or ectopic varices (10%) [29]. EHPVO more commonly results in IGV1 varices, whereas cirrhosis related portal hypertension more commonly results in GOV2 varices.

3.1 Primary prophylaxis

There is limited data on the primary prophylaxis of GV bleeding. In a RCT with a sample size of 89 patients, endoscopic glue was found to be more effective than the beta-blocker therapy in preventing the first GV bleeding, the risk of not having bleed, being 87% vs. 62% respectively. There was a survival advantage also in the patients with GOV2 and IGV1. High-risk factors for first bleeding from GVs are variceal size >20 mm, MELD score > 16, and the presence of severe portal hypertensive gastropathy (PHG) [31] and these may be suitable for glue injection. The algorithm for the management of gastric varix, including role of primary prophylaxis is depicted in **Figure 7**.

3.2 Acute gastric variceal hemorrhage (AGVH)

Medical management of suspected gastric variceal bleeding includes airway protection, restrictive blood transfusion, vasoactive agents, antibiotics, and admission to the intensive care unit. **Table 2** shows various modalities which can be used to treat GV. Endoscopic therapy is the initial treatment of choice. The methods utilized often depend on the local availability and experience. An algorithm for management of GV is shown in **Figure 7**.

3.3 Glue injection

N-butyl-2-cyanoacrylate, is a monomer that rapidly undergoes exothermic polymerization upon contact with living tissues, getting transformed from liquid to a hard, brittle acrylic plastic. This tissue adhesive is used to treat bleeding GV.

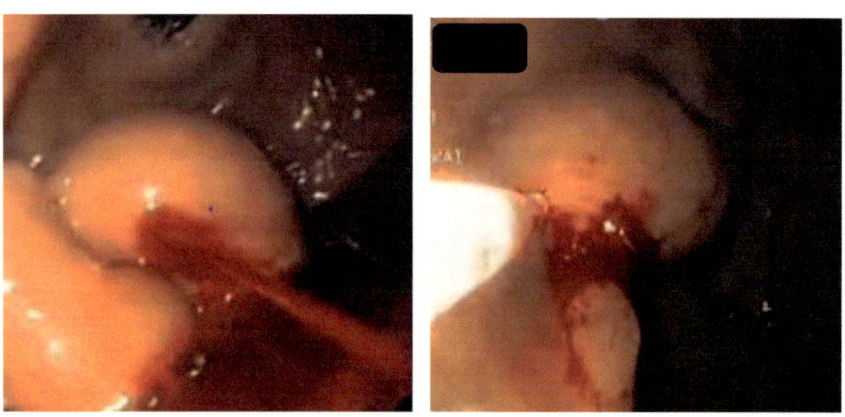

(a) (b)

Figure 6.
Endoscopic appearance of gastric varix. (a) Spurting bleeding from the gastric varix, (b) hemostasis after glue injection.

Endoscopic therapy
Glue
Coil
Thrombin
Sclerotherapy
Interventional Radiology
TIPS
BRTO/BATO
Surgery

Table 2.
Therapeutic options for control of acute gastric variceal bleed.

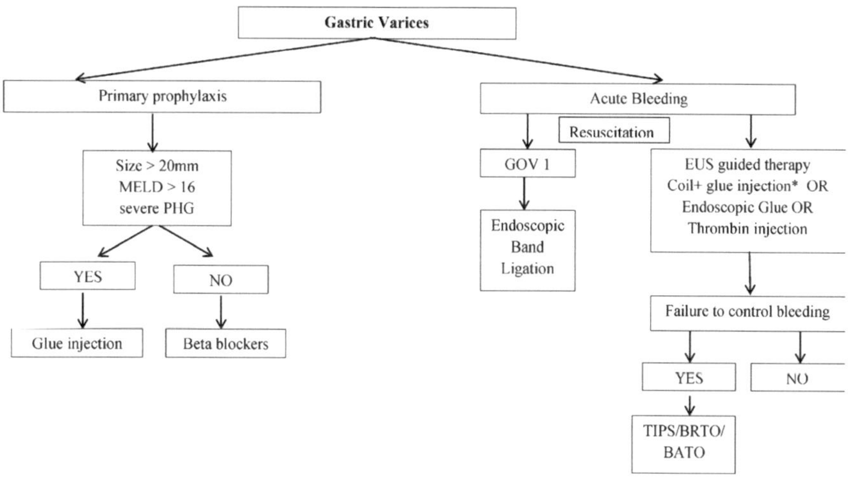

Figure 7.
Algorithm for management of gastric varix. Depending the expertise available. TIPS Transjugular intrahepatic portosystemic shunt. BRTO balloon-occluded retrograde transvenous obliteration. BATO balloon-occluded Antegrade Transvenous obliteration.

For the glue injection, a therapeutic endoscope with a 3.7 mm working channel may be preferred for the accurate control of the injector catheter. The injection catheter should be primed with distilled water (DW) or normal saline (NS) (0.8–1 ml) to fill up the dead space. The gastroscope is placed in a retroflexed position close to the target varix. The suction is turned off, and the injection catheter with the needle still withdrawn, is advanced without variceal contact juxtaposed to the target varix. The needle is then pushed out directly into the varix, and glue is injected in 1 ml aliquots by using NS or DW solution to flush the glue into the varix. The needle should be immediately withdrawn after the glue injection to prevent entrapment into the varix. While withdrawing the needle, the flushing of a steady stream of the solution is aimed at the varix's puncture site. The varix's blunt palpation is done by catheter or biopsy forceps, and additional glue is injected until the varix is 'hard' to palpate.

Overall success in term of hemostasis is noted in 84–100% of GV treated with glue. Technical complications related to glue injection include needle entrapment in a varix, exposure to the eyes of endoscopists or the assistants, or endoscope damage. Clinical complications from cyanoacrylate injection occur in up to 7% of cases and involve systemic embolization, sepsis, gastric ulcer, rebleeding due to cast extrusion, and mesenteric hematoma. Embolisation can be fatal and can involve lung, portal vein, coronary arteries, spleen, or even brain with risk increasing more with excessive and forceful glue injection. Visceral fistulization from the stomach into the pleura or mediastinum also may occur after unintentional paravariceal glue injection [32].

3.4 Sclerosant injection

Injection of sclerosants like tetradecyl sulphate and alcohol is one of the oldest techniques endoscopists used, in order to control acute gastric variceal bleeding. Sclerotherapy involves injection of a combination of para- and intra-variceal injections, or 5–10 ml of intravariceal sclerosant injection into the actively bleeding GV. Rebleeding rate is reported to be between 10 and 20%.

On comparing glue injection versus sclerotherapy in a RCT of 37 patients with IGV-1, glue was more efficacious than alcohol sclerotherapy in immediate hemostasis (89% vs. 62%), variceal obliteration (100% vs. 44%), and achieving quicker variceal obliteration (2 weeks vs. 4.7 weeks) [33]. Sclerosant injection is associated with high rates of complications, including gastric ulceration, perforation, and rebleeding (37–53%), and hence, it is not a good option in the management of GV [34, 35].

3.5 Thrombin injection

Thrombin tissue adhesives include thrombin, a human or bovine protein that affects hemostasis by converting fibrinogen to a fibrin clot. Thrombin also achieves hemostasis by altering the platelet aggregation. Human thrombin injection generally consists of 5 ml of reconstituted solution in calcium-chloride containing thrombin 500 IU/ml (Floseal; Baxter Healthcare Corporation, CA, Hayward, USA). During each session, usually 5 mL of thrombin solution is injected in a varix.

In an only RCT available which compares thrombin to cyanoacrylate injection in the control of AGVH, thrombin injection and glue injection had similar success rate (90% vs. 90.9%). However, a higher incidence of complications (51% vs. 12%) and ulcers (37% vs. 0%) were noted with glue injection as compared to thrombin [36]. Results of this study cannot be generalized as the sample size used in this study was small.

3.6 Endoscopic ultrasound (EUS) -guided therapies

EUS can improve the endoscopic management of gastric varices in many regards. These include – a) Increased detection rate of gastric varices overlooked as gastric folds. b) Ability to use doppler to confirm variceal obliteration and predicting the rebleeding risk. c) Adequate visualization of culprit gastric varix even in presence of torrential hemorrhage or blood clots and d) EUS-guided glue injection can be done precisely into a perforating vessel with preceding contrast injection to identify the feeding vessel as efferent or afferent, and thereby reducing embolization risk by enabling the use of a smaller volume of glue. e) EUS provides additional information regarding portal vein and splenic vein patency, helping to assess need and feasibility candidacy for TIPS/Balloon-occluded retrograde transvenous obliteration (BRTO) in failed cases [37].

The technique of EUS guided glue therapy involves filling the gastric fundus with water to improve acoustic coupling and visualization. The EUS is then positioned either in the distal esophagus (transesophageal-transcrural approach) or in the cardia/fundus (transgastric approach) to visualize the intramural varices and feeder vessels. EUS-directed intravascular puncture of the GV is performed using a standard FNA needle.

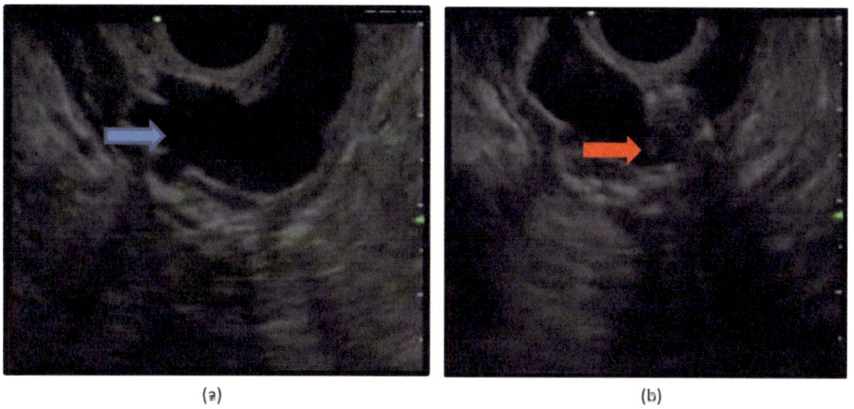

Figure 8.
Endosonographic coil embolization of the gastric varix. (a)Endosonography view of gastric varix (blue arrow) (b) Endosonography view of gastric varix after coil embolization(blue arrow).

Reports have suggested that the initial deployment of intravascular coils in the GV provides a scaffold for glue polymerization and fixation, reducing the glue requirement and inadvertent glue embolization [38] (**Figure 8**). Various commercially available coils include 0.035-inch MReye coils (extended embolus length 5 to 10 cm, coiled embolus diameter 10 mm; IMWCE 35, Cook Medical) or Hilal micro coils (extended embolus length 2 cm, coiled embolus diameter 2 mm; Embolization micro coil, MWCE, William Cook Europe, Bjeeverskov, DK). Generally, a 5-cm MReye coil are used if the vessel diameter is less than 10 mm, and a 10-cm MReye coil is used if the vessel diameter was more than 10 mm. Once the needle is inside the gastric varix, stylet is withdrawn, and the coil is deployed by advancing the stiffer part of a 0.035-inch guidewire. After coil is deployed, 1 ml aliquots of glue is injected, followed by NS flush, using the same needle. Color Doppler after treatment can confirm the absence of flow in the treated varix.

EUS-guided coil and cyanoacrylate injection was found to yield a 100% hemostatic success rate in a single-center pilot study [39]. Additionally, there were no procedure-related complications reported [39]. A recently published meta-analysis that compared treatment efficacy of EUS guided glue and coil injection with the endoscopic glue injection alone reported a statistically significant benefit of variceal obliteration in the EUS group (86.2% vs. 62.6%). The results were however, comparable in both the groups in terms of treatment efficacy, recurrence of gastric varix, early and late rebleeding [40].

3.7 Hemospray

TC-325 (Hemospray, Cook Medical, Winstom-Salem, North Carolina, United States) is a hemostatic powder which, when in contact with blood or tissue in the GI tract, becomes cohesive and adhesive, and forms a physical barrier, coating the bleeding site. Its effect lasts approximately 24 hours because the hemostatic layer sloughs off. Currently, it is only licensed for the treatment of non-variceal upper GI bleed. However, two recent studies demonstrated that Hemospray could be used as a bridge to a definitive treatment in active variceal bleeding [41, 42].

4. Ectopic varices

Ectopic varices (EcV) have a very complex anatomy. Understanding anastomosis with the splanchnic venous system is essential in managing EcV. These are rare

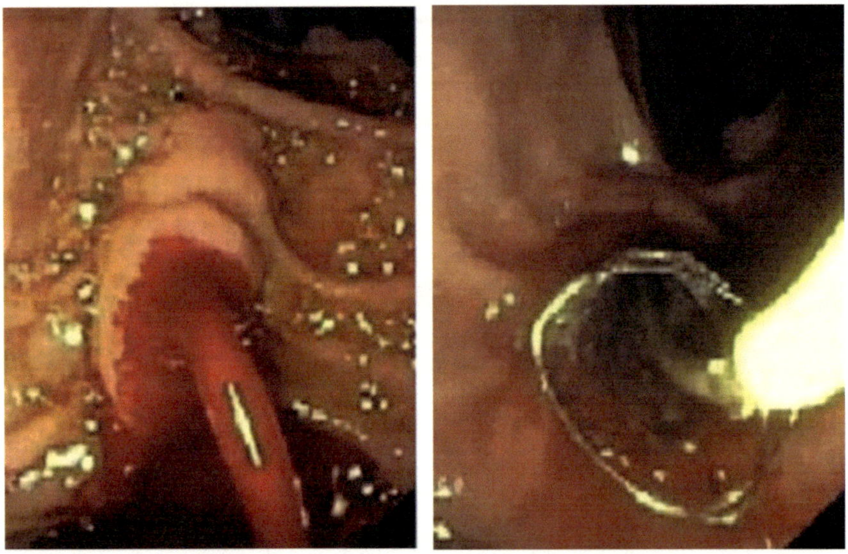
(a) (b)

Figure 9.
Hemobilia due to choledochal varix and its treatment with metal stent. (a) Endoscopic appearance at side viewing examination showing spurting from papilla due to choledochal varix, (b) after deployment of covered self-expanding metal stent.

cause of bleeding in patients with cirrhosis and PH, accounting for only 2–5% cases [43]. They are more common in patients with prehepatic PH, occurring in 27–40% of patients with splanchnic vein thrombosis [44]. However, EcV bleed is more severe than esophageal variceal bleeding, with mortality rates up to 37.5% [45]. Ectopic varix can develop in the duodenum, small bowel, rectum, colon, gallbladder, and biliary tract, periumbilical, peristomal, and the retroperitoneal areas. Endoscopy is used for both diagnosis and therapy. Most of the EcV are within reach of standard EGD and colonoscopy. A bleeding small intestinal varix may occasionally require the use of capsule endoscopy and device-assisted enteroscopy.

The treatment of bleeding of EcV is extrapolated from the esophageal and gastric varices literature. Successful outcomes depend on local expertise, location of varices, and the technical feasibility. ES and glue injection are commonly used modalities. EVL can be used to manage the rectal and duodenal varix. Caution however, must be exercised if the varix size is bigger, as the chances of hemostasis are less and the risk of rebleeding is high. Use of APC with EBL may be considered for the prevention of variceal occurrence, as has been reported in the treatment of ileocolonic anastomotic varices [45]. Hemostatic clip placement has been reported for ectopic variceal therapy [46]. Hemobilia, due to choledochal varices, can be life-threatening. Placement of a covered biliary metal stent (**Figure 9a**, **b**) is a promising approach to achieve immediate hemostasis for bleeding from portal biliopathy and associated choledochal varix. Biliary stenting serves as salvage therapy and a bridge to elective devascularization and shunt surgery [47].

5. Portal hypertensive gastropathy (PHG)

PHG, typically seen in patients with PH, is a condition of gastric mucosal ectasia and impaired mucosal defense. The incidence of PHG in patients with PH, varies greatly, ranging between 20 and 75%. Of those approximately 65–90%

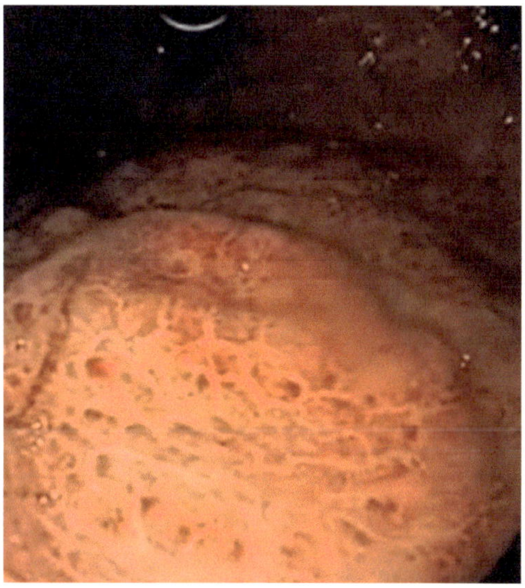

Figure 10
Severe portal hypertensive gastropathy.

have mild PHG (mosaic pattern of the gastric mucosa without red spots), whereas 10–25% have severe PHG (mosaic pattern of the gastric mucosa with red spots; **Figure 10**) [48]. The ectatic mucosal capillaries and venules of PHG may cause recurrent bleeding, presenting as acute or chronic occult blood loss. The annual incidence of overt bleeding from mild PHG is about 5%, while it is 15% for severe PHG [49]. The frequency of rebleeding of PHG is 11–30% [50].

APC has been evaluated for the treatment of PHG, in combination with adequate NSBB. This does reduce rates of blood transfusion, ICU admission, and improve hemoglobin levels in 80–90% of patients [51, 52]. Hemospray is also an option for the treatment of active PHG bleeding. However, these endoscopic methods may be an effective bridging therapy till TIPS or liver transplant is performed [53].

6. Gastric antral vascular ectasia (GAVE)

GAVE is characterized by erythematous or raised mucosa with underlying tortuous ectatic vessels as red spots. Patterns of GAVE include honeycombing, diffuse or speckled patchy erythema, and nodular antral GAVE. These appear as diffuse or linear array in the gastric antrum **(Figure 11a)**. Both PHG and GAVE may be found during endoscopy in patients with PH or discovered during variceal screening. However, in most instances, they are distinguished by their endoscopic appearance, location and when needed, biopsy for histological examination. (**Table 3**). On histology, GAVE shows presence of fibromuscular hyperplasia, fibrin microthrombi, and increased neuroendocrine cells in the lamina propria [54]. GAVE can be isolated or can be associated with cirrhosis and with systemic illnesses like scleroderma, chronic renal failure, and can occur after bone marrow transplantation. PH does not play a direct role in development of GAVE, as it is not present in up to 70% of patients, and the reduction of portal hypertension does not affect the course of the disease [55].

The endoscopic treatment includes laser photoablation, APC, radio-frequency ablation [56], EVL, and cryotherapy. APC is the most common, efficacious, and feasible therapeutic option for the treatment of GAVE **(Figure 11b),** with a reported efficacy of 90%- 100% causing a significant reduction in blood

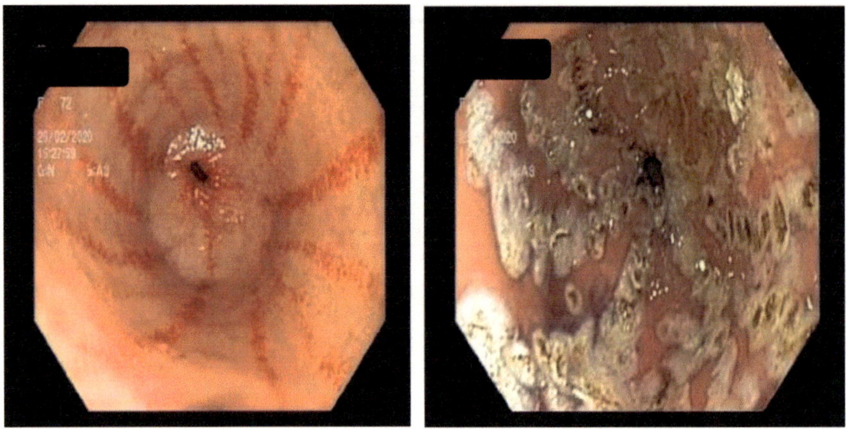

(a) (b)

Figure 11.
Endoscopic appearance of gastric antral vascular ectasia. (a) Endoscopic appearance of gastric antral vascular ectasia, (b) appearance after argon plasma coagulation.

			Portal Hypertensive Gastropathy	**Gastric Antral Vascular Ectasia**
1.	Definition		PHG, typically seen in patients with PH, is a condition of gastric mucosal ectasia and impaired mucosal defense	It is characterized by erythematous or raised mucosa with underlying tortuous ectatic vessels as red spots in either a diffuse or linear array
2.	Location		Gastric fundus and body	Gastric antrum
3.	Association with Portal HTN		Always	In approximately 30% case
4.	Histology		Dliated mucosal and submucosal veins along with ectatic capillaries without microthrombi or inflammation	Fibromuscular hyperplasia, fibrin microthrombi, and increased neuroendocrine cells in the lamina propria
5.	Endoscopy		Mosaic pattern (mild) with red spots (severe)	Honeycombing, Diffuse or speckled patchy erythema, and nodular antral lesions
6.	Incidence of bleed		Low	Higher than PHG related bleed
7.	Treatment	First line	NSBB	EBL Thermocoagulation
		Second line	Thermocoagulation Liver transplantation	Cryotherapy Radiofrequency ablation Anterectomy

Table 3.
Difference between portal hypertensive Gastropathy and gastric antral vascular ectasia.

transfusion requirement [57, 58]. The setting of argon gas flow usually ranges between 0.8–2.0 L/min, the electrical power from 40 to 60 W, and, generally, a mean of 2.5 sessions are needed to achieve complete eradication [59]. Few studies have compared EVL with APC for GAVE treatment, where band ligation showed a significantly higher rate of hemostasis, required fewer treatment sessions, a higher increase in hemoglobin values, and reduced need for blood transfusions [60, 61]. The higher efficacy EVL is attributed to a more controlled and reliable eradication of the abnormal vasculature in the mucosa and submucosa.

7. Portal hypertensive enteropathy (PHE)

PHE is a condition associated with pathologic changes and mucosal abnormalities in the small intestine of patients with PH. It is being increasingly diagnosed, due to the advent of video capsule endoscopy and deep enteroscopy. In recent studies, the prevalence of PHE varies around 93–97%, with 8–12% of patients showing evidence of ongoing bleeding [62–64]. The findings of PHE are characterized as vascular (red spots, telangiectasia, or varices) and non-vascular or inflammatory (villous edema, erythema, or polyps) changes [64] (**Figure 12a-f**).

Treatment options for PHE related bleed include glue or sclerosant for variceal bleeding and APC for non-variceal bleeding. In patients with hemodynamic instability, radiological coil embolization is an option [64].

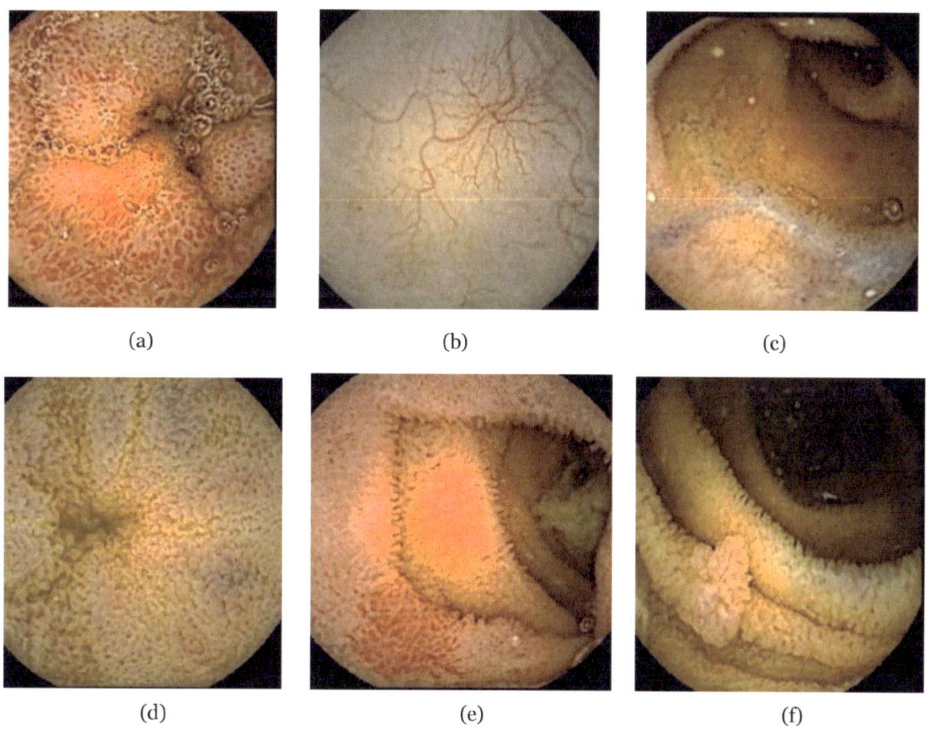

Figure 12.
Capsule endoscopy appearance of portal hypertensive enteropathy. a-c: Vascular: (a) red spot, (b) telangiectasia, (c) small intestinal varix. d-e: Inflammatory: (d) villous edema, (e) erythema, (f) polyp.

8. Portal hypertensive COLOPATHY (PHC)

Colonic abnormalities in patients with PH are referred to as PHC, and these are vascular ectasias, mosaic pattern mucosa, mucosal hemorrhages, anorectal or colonic varices, hemorrhoids, and nonspecific inflammatory changes. Its prevalence in patients with cirrhosis varies from 25 to 70%, with an estimated bleeding rate of 0–9% [65–68]. Treatment options are ES or glue injection for variceal bleed, EVL for hemorrhoidal bleed, and APC for the non-variceal bleed and are similar to those in PHE.

9. Summary

PH can result in formation of varices at various sites with mucosal changes anywhere in the gastrointestinal tract. These can lead to acute gastrointestinal bleed or anemia. Endoscopy plays an important role in diagnosis and treatment of these complications. EVL and glue are the usual first line treatment for esophageal and GV respectively. Other therapies include sclerosant or thrombin injection, EUS-guided therapies, esophageal stent placement, APC or hemospray.

Author details

Bhavik Bharat Shah, Usha Goenka and Mahesh Kumar Goenka*
Apollo Gleneagles Hospitals, Kolkata, India

*Address all correspondence to: mkgkolkata@gmail.com

References

[1] Sharma M, Rameshbabu CS. Collateral pathways in portal hypertension. J Clin Exp Hepatol 2012;2(4): 338-52.

[2] Thuluvath PJ, Yoo HY. Portal hypertensive gastropathy. Am J Gastroenterol 2002 Dec 1;97(12):2973-8.

[3] D'Amico G, Pagliaro L, Bosch J. The treatment of portal hypertension: a meta-analytic review. Hepatology 1995; 22: 332-354.

[4] Garcia-Tsao G, Abraldes JG, Berzigotti A, et al. Portal hypertensive bleeding in cirrhosis: Risk stratification, diagnosis, and management: 2016 practice guidance by the American Association for the study of liver diseases. Hepatology 2017;65(1):310-35.

[5] D'Amico G, Pasta L, Morabito A, et al. Competing risks and prognostic stages of cirrhosis: a 25-year inception cohort study of 494 patients. Aliment Pharmacol Ther 2014;39:1180-1193.

[6] Augustin S, Muntaner L, Altamirano JT, et al. Predicting early mortality after acute variceal hemorrhage based on classification and regression tree analysis. Clin Gastroenterol Hepatol 2009;7:1347-1354.

[7] Bosch J, García-Pagán JC. Prevention of variceal rebleeding. Lancet. 2003 Mar 15;361(9361):952-4.

[8] de Franchis R, Eisen GM, Laine L, et al. Esophageal capsule endoscopy for screening and surveillance of esophageal varices in patients with portal hypertension. Hepatology. 2008;47:1595-1603.

[9] Wang HM, Lo GH, Chen WC, et al. Efficacy of transient elastography in screening for large esophageal varices in patients with suspicious or proven liver cirrhosis. J Dig Dis. 2012;13:430-438.

[10] North Italian Endoscopic Club for the Study and Treatment of Esophageal Varices. Prediction of the first variceal hemorrhage in patients with cirrhosis of the liver and esophageal varices. A prospective multicenter study. N Engl J Med 1988; 319: 983-989

[11] European Association for the Study of the Liver. EASL Clinical Practice Guidelines for the management of patients with decompensated cirrhosis. J. Hepatol. 2018 Aug 1;69(2):406-60.

[12] Kapoor A, Dharel N, Sanyal AJ. Endoscopic diagnosis and therapy in gastroesophageal variceal bleeding. Gastrointest Endosc Clin N Am 2015;25(3):491-507.

[13] De Franchis R Baveno VI faculty. Expanding consensus in portal hypertension: report of the BAVENO VI Consensus Workshop: Stratifying risk and individualizing care for portal hypertension. J Hepatol 2015;63:743-752.

[14] Garcia-Tsao G, Sanyal AJ, Grace ND, Carey W. Practice Guidelines Committee of the American Association for the Study of Liver Diseases Practice Parameters Committee of the American College of Gastroenterology. Prevention and management of gastroesophageal varices and variceal hemorrhage in cirrhosis. Hepatology 2007;46:922-938.

[15] D'Amico G, De Franchis R. Upper digestive bleeding in cirrhosis. Post-therapeutic outcome and prognostic indicators. Hepatology 2003; 38: 599-612.

[16] Villanueva C, Colomo A, Bosch A, et al. Transfusion strategies for acute upper gastrointestinal bleeding. N Engl J Med 2013;368:11 21.

[17] Avgerinos A, Armonis A, Stefanidis G, et al. Sustained rise of portal pressure after sclerotherapy, but not band ligation, in acute variceal bleeding in cirrhosis. Hepatology 2004; 39:1623-1630.

[18] Garcia-Tsao G, Abraldes JG, Berzigotti A, Bosch J. Portal hypertensive bleeding in cirrhosis: Risk stratification, diagnosis, and management 2016 practice guidance by the American Association for the study of liver diseases. Hepatology 2017;65:310-335.

[19] Dai C, Liu WX, Jiang M, et al. Endoscopic variceal ligation compared with endoscopic injection sclerotherapy for treatment of esophageal variceal hemorrhage: a meta-analysis. World J Gastroenterol 2015;21(8):2534-41.

[20] Kapoor A, Dharel N, Sanyal AJ. Endoscopic diagnosis and therapy in gastroesophageal variceal bleeding. Gastrointest Endosc Clin N Am 2015;25(3): 491-507.

[21] Maluf-Filho F, Sakai P, Ishioka S, et al. Endoscopic sclerosis versus cyanoacrylate endoscopic injection for the first episode of variceal bleeding: a prospective, controlled, and randomized study in Child-Pugh class C patients. Endoscopy 2001;33(5):421-7.

[22] Azoulay D, Castaing D, Majno P, et al. Salvage transjugular intrahepatic portosystemic shunt for uncontrolled variceal bleeding in patients with decompensated cirrhosis. J Hepatol. 2001;35:590-7.

[23] Chesta FN, Rizvi ZH, Oberoi M, Buttar N. The role of stenting in patients with variceal bleeding. Techniques and Innovations in Gastrointestinal Endoscopy. 2020 Jul 23 (In press).

[24] Goenka MK, Goenka U, Tiwary IK, Rai V. Use of self-expanding metal stents for difficult variceal bleed. Indian J Gastroenterol. 2017 Nov 1;36(6):468-73.

[25] McCarty TR, Njei B: Self-expanding metal stents for acute refractory esophageal variceal bleeding: A systematic review and meta-analysis. Dig Endosc 2016, 28(5):539-547.

[26] Maufa F, Al-Kawas FH: Role of self-expandable metal stents in acute variceal bleeding. Int J Hepatol 2012, 2012:418369-418369.

[27] Kamal A, Abd Elmoety AA, Hamza Y, Zeid A. Endoscopic variceal ligation followed by argon plasma coagulation against endoscopic variceal ligation alone. J Clin Gastroenterol. 2017 Jan 1;51(1):49-55.

[28] Li X, Jiang T, Gao J. Endoscopic variceal ligation combined with argon plasma coagulation versus ligation alone for the secondary prophylaxis of variceal bleeding: a systematic review and meta-analysis. Eur J Gastroenterol Hepatol 2017;29(6):621-8.

[29] Sarin SK, Lahoti D, Saxena SP, et al. Prevalence, classification and natural history of gastric varices: a long-term follow-up study in 568 portal hypertension patients. Hepatology 1992;16:1343-1349.

[30] de Franchis R, Primignani M. Natural history of portal hypertension in patients with cirrhosis. Clin Liver Dis 2001; 5: 645-63.

[31] Mishra SR, Sharma BC, Kumar A, Sarin SK. Primary prophylaxis of gastric variceal bleeding comparing cyanoacrylate injection and beta-blockers: a randomized controlled trial. J Hepatol 2011; 54: 1161-1167.

[32] Tripathi D, Ferguson JW, Therapondos G, Plevris JN, Hayes PC. Recent advances in the management of bleeding gastric varices Aliment. Pharmacol. Ther. 2006 Jul;24(1):1-7.

[33] Sarin SK, Jain AK, Jain M, Gupta R. A randomized controlled trial of cyanoacrylate versus alcohol injection in patients with isolated fundic varices. Am J Gastroenterol. 2002;97(4):1010-5.

[34] Sarin SK. Long-term follow-up of gastric variceal sclerotherapy: an eleven year experience. Gastrointest Endosc 1997; 46: 8-14.

[35] Trudeau W, Prindiville T. Endoscopic injection sclerosis in bleeding gastric varices. Gastrointest Endosc 1986;32(4):264-8.

[36] Lo GH, Lin CW, Tai CM, et al. A prospective, randomized trial of thrombin versus cyanoacrylate injection in the control of acute gastric variceal hemorrhage. Endoscopy. 2020.

[37] Nett A, Binmoeller KF. Endoscopic Management of Portal Hypertension–related Bleeding Gastrointest Endoscopy Clin N Am 29 (2019) 321-337.

[38] Weilert F, Binmoeller KF. Endoscopic management of gastric variceal bleeding. Gastroenterol Clin North Am 2014;43(4):807-18.

[39] Binmoeller KF, Weilert F, Shah JN, Kim J. EUS-guided transesophageal treatment of gastric fundal varices with combined coiling and cyanoacrylate glue injection (with videos). Gastrointest Endosc. 2011;74:1019-25.

[40] Mohan BP, Chandan S, Khan SR, et al. Efficacy and safety of endoscopic ultrasound-guided therapy versus direct endoscopic glue injection therapy for gastric varices: systematic review and meta-analysis. Endoscopy. 2020;52(4):259-67.

[41] HolIbrahim M, El-Mikkawy A, Hamid MA, et al. Early application of haemostatic powder added to standard management for oesophagogastric variceal bleeding: a randomised trial. Gut. 2019 1;68(5):844-53.

[42] Holster IL, Poley JW, Kuipers EJ, Tjwa ET. Controlling gastric variceal bleeding with endoscopically applied hemostatic powder (Hemospray™). J Hepatol 2012; 57: 1397-1398.

[43] Henry Z, Uppal D, Saad W, et al. Gastric and ectopic varices. Clin Liver Dis 2014;18:371-88.

[44] Orr DW, Harrison PM, Devlin J, et al. Chronic mesenteric venous thrombosis: evaluation and determinants of survival during long-term follow-up. Clin Gastroenterol Hepatol 2007;5(1):80-6.

[45] Helmy A, Al Kahtani K, Al Fadda M. Updates in the pathogenesis, diagnosis and management of ectopic varices. Hepatol Int 2008;2(3):322-34.

[46] Park SW, Cho E, Jun CH, et al. Upper gastrointestinal ectopic variceal bleeding treated with various endoscopic modalities: case reports and literature review. Medicine (Baltimore) 2017;96(1):e5860.

[47] Goenka MK, Harwani Y, Rai V, Goenka U. Fully covered self-expandable metal biliary stent for hemobilia caused by portal biliopathy. Gastrointest Endosc. 2014 Dec 1;80(6):1175.

[48] Merli M, Nicolini G, Angeloni S, Gentili F, Attili AF, Riggio O. The natural history of portal hypertensive gastropathy in patients with liver cirrhosis and mild portal hypertension. Am J Gastroenterol. 2004;**99**:1959-654.

[49] D'Amico G, Garcia-Tsao G, Pagliaro L. Natural history and prognostic indicators of survival in cirrhosis: a systematic review of 118 studies. J Hepatol 2006; 44: 217-231.

[50] Primignani M, Carpinelli L, Preatoni P et al. Portal hypertensive gastropathy (PHG) in liver cirrhosis: natural history. A multicenter study by the New Italian Endoscopic Club (NIEC). J Gastroenterol 1996; 110: 1299.

[51] Herrera S, Bordas JM, Liach J et al. The beneficial effects of argon plasma coagulation in the management of different types of gastric vascular ectasia lesions in patients admitted for GI hemorrhage. Gastrointest Endosc 2008; 68: 440-446.

[52] Hanafy AS, El Hawary AT. Efficacy of argon plasma coagulation in the management of portal hypertensive

gastropathy. Endosc Int Open 2016;4(10):E1057-62.

[53] Smith LA, Morris AJ, Stanley AJ. The use of hemospray in portal hypertensive bleeding; a case series. J Hepatol 2014;60(2):457-60.

[54] Burak KW, Lee SS, Beck PL. Portal hypertensive gastropathy and gastric antral vascular ectasia (GAVE) syndrome. Gut 2001; 49: 866-872.

[55] Spahr L, Villeneuve JP, Dufresne MP, et al. Gastric antral vascular ectasia in cirrhotic patients: absence of relation with portal hypertension. Gut 1999; 44: 739-742.

[56] Thandassery RB, Jha AK, Goenka MK. Gastrointestinal radiofrequency ablation in the management of refractory gastric antral vascular eclasia. J Gastroenterol hepatol 2014; 29: 894

[57] Roman S, Saurin JC, Dumortier J, Perreira A, Bernard G, Ponchon T. Tolerance and efficacy of argon plasma coagulation for controlling bleeding in patients with typical and atypical manifestations of watermelon stomach. Endoscopy 2003; 35: 1024-1028.

[58] Yusoff I, Brennan F, Ormonde D, Laurence B. Argon plasma coagulation for treatment of watermelon stomach. Endoscopy 2002; 34: 407-410.

[59] Sebastian S, McLoughlin R, Qasim A, O'Morain CA, Buckley MJ. Endoscopic argon plasma coagulation for the treatment of gastric antral vascular ectasia (watermelon stomach): long-term results. Dig Liver Dis 2004; 36: 212-217.

[60] Wells CD, Harrison ME, Gurudu SR, Crowell MD, Byrne TJ, Depetris G, Sharma VK. Treatment of gastric antral vascular ectasia (watermelon stomach) with endoscopic band ligation. Gastrointest Endosc 2008; 68: 231-236.

[61] Elhendawy M, Mosaad S, Alkhalawany W, Abo-Ali L, Enaba M, Elsaka A, Elfert AA. Randomized controlled study of endoscopic band ligation and argon plasma coagulation in the treatment of gastric antral and fundal vascular ectasia. United European Gastroenterol. J.. 2016 Jun;4(3):423-8.

[62] Chandrasekar TS, Janakan GB, Chandrasekar VT, Kalamegam RY, Suriyanarayanan S, Sanjeevaraya PM. Spectrum of small-bowel mucosal identified by capsule endoscopy in patients with portal hypertension of varied etiology. Indian J Gastroenterol 2017;36:32-37.

[63] Akyuz F, Pinarbasi B, Ermis F, et al. Is portal hypertensive enteropathy an important additional cause of blood loss in portal hypertensive patients? J Gastroenterol 2010;45:1497-1502.

[64] Goenka MK, Shah BB, Rai VK, Jajodia S, Goenka U. Mucosal changes in the small intestines in portal hypertension: first study using the Pillcam SB3 capsule endoscopy system. Clin Endosc. 2018 Nov;51(6):563.

[65] Bresci G, Parisi G, Capria A. Clinical relevance of colonic lesions in cirrhotic patients with portal hypertension. Endoscopy. 2006; 38:830-5.

[66] Rabinovitz M, Schade RR, Dindzans VJ, et al. Colonic disease in cirrhosis. An endoscopic evaluation in 412 patients. Gastroenterology. 1990; 99:195-9.

[67] Chen LS, Lin HC, Lee FY, et al. Portal hypertensive colopathy in patients with cirrhosis. Scand J Gastroenterol. 1996; 31:490-4.

[68] Goenka M K, Kochhar R, Nagi B, Mehta S K. Rectosigmoid varices and other mucosal changes in patients with portal hypertension. Am J Gastroenterol 1991; 86 : 1185-9.